Which Tests
for My
Unborn Baby?

Which Tests for My Unborn Baby?

ULTRASOUND AND OTHER PRENATAL TESTS

LACHLAN DE CRESPIGNY

**with
RHONDA DREDGE**

NEW EDITION

Melbourne

OXFORD UNIVERSITY PRESS

Oxford Auckland New York

OXFORD UNIVERSITY PRESS AUSTRALIA
Oxford   New York
Athens   Auckland   Bangkok   Bombay
Calcutta   Cape Town   Dar es Salaam   Delhi
Florence   Hong Kong   Istanbul   Karachi
Kuala Lumpur   Madras   Madrid   Melbourne
Mexico City   Nairobi Paris   Port Moresby   Singapore
Taipei   Tokyo   Toronto
and associated companies in
Berlin   Ibadan

OXFORD is a trade mark of Oxford University Press

Copyright © Lachlan de Crespigny with Rhonda Dredge 1991, 1996
First published 1991
Revised edition 1996
Reprinted 1997

National Library of Australia
Cataloguing-in-Publication data:

de Crespigny, Lachlan James Champion.
Which tests for my unborn baby?: ultrasound
and other prenatal tests.

   2nd ed.
   Includes index.
   ISBN 0 19 553954 0.

   1. Prenatal diagnosis – Popular works. 2. Ultrasonics in
   obstetrics – Popular works. 3. Fetal monitoring – Popular
   works. I. Dredge, Rhonda, II. Title.

   618.32075

Cover design by Cath Lindsey
Text design by Kirstin Lowe
Cover picture: Australian Picture Library
Illustrations by Juli Kent
Typeset by Supagraphics, Collingwood, Victoria
Printed through Bookpac Production Services, Singapore
Published by Oxford University Press,
253 Normanby Road, South Melbourne, Australia.

contents

To Margaret,
wife, colleague and friend

I wish to thank my many colleagues and friends who read part or all of the first edition of this book. I especially wish to thank Dr Eric Haan, Dr John Hobbins, Dr Hugh Robinson, Dr George Kossoff and Professor Roger Pepperell. I am also indebted to the cytogenetic department at the Royal Women's Hospital for the two karyograms and Dr Marjorie England and Wolfe Publications for allowing me to use the anatomical pictures in figure 1.1. I am grateful to Ms Lou Sweetland from Oxford University Press without whose enthusiasm this book would not have begun.

L. C.
1991

I wish to thank the Murdoch Institute for Research into Birth Defects and Ann Robertson at the Royal Women's Hospital for their expert guidance on genetic counselling. Paramount, though, is my appreciation of the many women who willingly shared their experiences of prenatal diagnosis.

R. D.

Acknowledgments

In the five years since the first edition of this book was published, no new tests have been introduced. Yet our understanding of the available tests, and the sophistication of their analysis, has changed dramatically. Serum screening, a method of testing a pregnant woman's blood to determine her risk of carrying a fetus with Down syndrome, is now widely used. Subtle variations visible on ultrasound are now better understood. For example, the presence of nuchal oedema, a soft tissue swelling at the back of the neck, has been found to be a much more important sign of Down syndrome than was realised in 1991. These techniques, which involve no risk to the fetus, can now be used as screening tests for Down syndrome, instead of the more invasive procedures.

Fetal medicine is now an established medical specialty, and the practice and ethics of prenatal diagnosis have continued to be a prominent area of debate within society. A study suggesting that the quality of ultrasound services available to Australian women was less than optimal recently made front-page news. More than 95 per cent of fetuses with spina bifida should be detected by ultrasound performed between 18 and 20 weeks. However, statewide studies suggest that up to 40 per cent of these abnormalities are being missed. Many more couples are asking obstetricians and those providing ultrasound services penetrating questions about the availability and quality of the tests. Such consumer interest can only be applauded. Medical services should be subject to the same consumer scrutiny as any other service.

Discussion of these issues demands careful use of terminology. In this new edition, the words *baby* and *mother* have been replaced, where appropriate, by the terms *fetus* and *pregnant woman*. The terms *mother* and *pregnant woman* are often used interchangeably, although their meanings are not identical. In general usage, a 'mother' is a female parent, one who has borne a child — the term therefore does not apply to a pregnant woman. In most Western countries a pregnant woman has a right to an abortion in certain circumstances. This contrasts with the ethical and legal responsibilities that a mother and father have towards their child. Clearly, to use the words *baby* and *fetus* interchangeably implies that they are of equal legal status, although in many States of Australia there is no legal limit on the gestational age for termination of pregnancy. In the instances where major congenital abnormalities are diagnosed through prenatal testing, couples can face extremely painful decisions regarding the future of the pregnancy. The terminology used in this field is important in assisting women and their partners in making decisions under great stress, and in respecting the different ethical and legal positions of fetus and baby, pregnant woman and mother.

This book does not present arguments for and against prenatal testing. It is written for the individual women and couples facing their own decisions. In chapter 10, we discuss the ways in which diagnostic tests are different from most other medical tests. Decisions about which tests are right for you cannot be made by doctors; they must be made on personal grounds, including your religious and moral beliefs, and the desires and expectations of your family. There is a new focus in medicine on caring for individual needs, and health professionals now expect that patients will ask questions about the services available. This is a welcome change. In the past, the prime concern of doctors was often the technology and its role in detecting abnormalities. However, women take part in prenatal testing to ensure that their babies will be healthy, and these services should be provided in a caring environment.

Without adequate information about the tests, pregnant women are not able to ask appropriate questions. This book aims to provide that information. The new edition includes a major expansion of many sections, particularly those on no-risk testing, ethical issues, and counselling. Despite the advances, prenatal diagnostic tests do not magically prevent birth defects. It is estimated, for example, that one in 200 infants is born with an intellectual disability. Chromosome abnormalities, the major reason for testing, account for only around 40 per cent of these. There are many other disorders, some environmental, some genetic, that no currently available test can diagnose.

At their best, however, prenatal tests can be life-saving. Ultrasound can forewarn of the existence of some rare conditions that require urgent medical attention at birth. The genetic tests are also extremely useful for women at higher risk of delivering a child with certain birth defects. The chances of a woman delivering a child with a chromosomal disorder begin to rise at 30 years of age and accelerate after 35. Prenatal diagnosis gives these women the chance to exclude some of the uncertainties and anxieties surrounding pregnancy.

Invasive tests usually rely on removing and analysing amniotic fluid or cells from the developing placenta. There are undoubted, although small, risks of the tests causing a miscarriage, so they are not routine procedures in all pregnancies. The perception of the risks involved also varies according to the situation; if a woman has already experienced several miscarriages, a stillborn baby, a sudden infant death, or a long period of infertility, any risk may be seen as threatening.

This book examines the issues vital to the emotional health of pregnant women and their families, as well as providing an account of the range of procedures available. As in any skilled field, however, the expertise of operators performing ultrasound and genetic tests varies. Results and risks quoted in this book assume that state-of-the-art equipment is used by experienced and skilled operators. Chapter 10 includes guidelines to help you assess whether you are receiving maximum care and safety.

You may not wish to read this book from cover to cover but to select the chapters important to you. If you are less than thirty-five years old, and have had no previous baby with spina bifida or chromosome abnormalities, chapters 1 to 4, which cover ultrasound, and chapter 8, which covers other non-invasive tests, will be most relevant. If you are over thirty-five, read the chapters on amniocentesis and chorionic villus sampling as well. A number of commonly asked questions are answered at the end of each chapter.

If you are concerned about the relationship between doctor and patient, chapter 9 covers the ethical issues involved, and if you are having trouble deciding whether testing is appropriate for you, the experiences of others outlined in chapter 10 may help. The increased understanding of prenatal tests does have its down side — it is now more difficult than ever for pregnant women to decide which tests they should have. Chapter 12 provides an easy reference by summarising the medical features of the available tests.

Normal Fetal Development

To understand the tests available in pregnancy you need to have some knowledge of the fundamentals of healthy pregnancy. This chapter highlights the normal development of the fetus, including discussion of the major milestones such as conception, the beginning of fetal movement, the development and normal function of the major organs, and the importance of the placenta and amniotic fluid to the well-being of the fetus.

One of the most satisfying things about performing an ultrasound examination is observing the pleasure couples gain from seeing the fetus on the screen. Most are stunned that it is so human-like, as early as 10 weeks. 'Look, it's moving already.' 'I can see its arms.' 'Is its heart already beating?' These are typical of the comments an ultrasound operator will hear every day. They are also indicative of the general lack of knowledge within the community about early fetal development. Most people are surprised at just how quickly the fetus develops from a single cell. Before covering the technique of ultrasound in depth, therefore, we will describe fetal development and relate this to what you will see on the ultrasound screen.

TIME OF CONCEPTION

On average, conception occurs around 14 days after the first day of the last menstrual period, i.e. in the middle of the next cycle. While most women know the date their last menstrual period began, very few can be certain when they conceived unless they were having special investigations as part of treatment for infertility. In obstetrics it is therefore not possible to use the real date of commencement of pregnancy and for convenience the pregnancy is said to begin on the first day of the last menstrual period.

EARLY DEVELOPMENT

It is extraordinary just how quickly the fetus develops. It changes from a single cell two weeks after the last period began to having a very human appearance eight weeks later. A fetus has fully formed arms, legs, face, head and body at 11 weeks after the last menstrual period began (see figure 1.1). From 11 weeks until delivery is a time of growth and maturation, most of the basic structures already being fully formed (see table 1.1).

From a medical viewpoint, knowing the timing of fetal development is important in assessing the possible impact of teratogens. This is a general term for substances such as Thalidomide, or viruses such as rubella (German measles), which can damage the fetus during a particular period of its development. Babies who were born with an abnormality of the arms or legs due to Thalidomide, for example, must have been exposed to the drug when they were developing between 5 and 9 weeks. Similarly, a baby with spina bifida, a condition in which the spinal canal does not fully close, shows defective development prior to 6 weeks when the spine is forming.

MOVEMENTS

Pregnant women are amazed to see the fetus moving on ultrasound at 8 to 9 weeks as they are unable to feel the movements until around 18 to 20 weeks, or sometimes a little earlier in second and subsequent

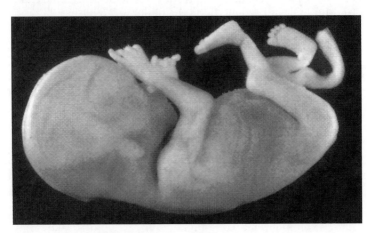

Figure 1.1 A normal fetus at 10–11 weeks.

TABLE 1.1 MAJOR EVENTS IN PREGNANCY

Gestation (weeks)	Milestone
0	1st day last menstrual period
2	Release of egg (ovulation)
4	
6	
8	Movements begin
10	CVS performed
12	
14	
16	Amniocentesis performed
18	Ultrasound to check fetal development
20	Movements usually felt
22	
24	Babies delivered have a reasonable prospect of survival
26	
28	
30	
32	
34	Babies delivered unlikely to have serious complications due to prematurity
36	
38	

40 (9 months + 7 days) due date

pregnancies. The woman will only start to feel movements when the fetus is strong enough to kick hard against her abdominal wall. Even after the onset of movements (quickening) only a small proportion of them are felt. When ultrasound shows a vigorously moving fetus late in pregnancy, you still may feel nothing, and may not do so for many days. This situation is actually a blessing — to be aware of each movement from 8 weeks until delivery would be exhausting.

THE PLACENTA

The pregnancy becomes attached to the wall of the uterus on day 20, six days after fertilization. Once attached, the very early placenta — the chorion — starts to function to provide oxygen and nutrients to the fetus and to remove wastes.

Until 8 weeks the chorion appears on the ultrasound screen as a thick white layer totally surrounding the fetus (see figure 1.2). In the early weeks of pregnancy you therefore cannot tell where the placenta will develop. At 9 weeks the chorion begins to thicken in one area while thinning elsewhere. By 10 weeks it is clearly seen on one wall of the uterus (see figure 1.3) and is now called the placenta rather than the chorion. The chorion is made up of cells derived from the fetus. It is these that are tested in chorionic villus sampling (CVS).

The early placenta has enormous reserves and powers of regeneration. Even if it becomes partially separated from the uterine wall by a blood clot it can recover and a healthy baby result. Even late in pregnancy there is enough reserve for the fetus to survive if half or more of the placenta separates.

The exchange across the placenta occurs without any mixing of blood between the pregnant woman and the fetus (see figure 1.4). They are totally separated by a thin membrane, although at times small amounts of fetal blood can cross into the woman's circulation. (In the same way, non-identical twins with a single placenta have separate circulations, each using its own half of the placenta independently. Identical twins, however, usually do have some communication between their circulations.)

At any stage of pregnancy it is not important how the placenta looks on ultrasound but rather how well it functions. Many fetuses have died with a placenta that looks absolutely normal. Ways of testing its function include looking at the growth of the fetus, its well-being and the amount of amniotic fluid present. The texture of the placenta itself is usually immaterial.

GROWTH

Every pregnant woman is anxious to find out whether the fetus is growing normally, particularly if a previous baby was especially large or small, if there has been a complication such as bleeding, or if they feel or look small compared to others at a similar stage. In fact, in the

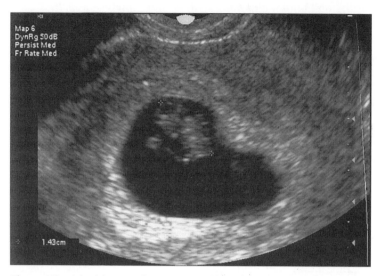

Figure 1.2 A healthy 7-week pregnancy. Within the sac, the fetus lies between the crosses with its head at the top left. The white rim (the chorion) surrounds the pregnancy sac. The dots on the right are half centimetres.

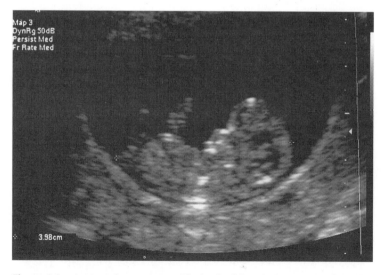

Figure 1.3 A 10-week pregnancy with the fetal face looking up on the right. The cord is visible as it enters the abdomen, and one of the legs in bent up in front of the abdomen.

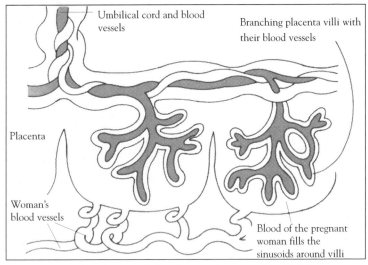

Umbilical cord and blood vessels

Branching placenta villi with their blood vessels

Placenta

Woman's blood vessels

Blood of the pregnant woman fills the sinusoids around villi

Figure 1.4 As this diagram of the placenta shows, the blood of the pregnant woman and the fetus does not mix, but exchange of nutrition and waste occurs across the villi. Blood from the cord passes through the villi, which are surrounded by the pregnant woman's blood in cavities called sinusoids.

first half of pregnancy, all fetuses grow at much the same rate. Measuring parts of the fetus such as its overall length or head size can therefore reliably show the degree of advancement of the pregnancy. If growth falls behind the expected rate prior to 20 weeks it may mean dire consequences for the fetus, but these circumstances are rare.

Table 1.2 summarizes the sequential development of the fetus and indicates its approximate length, weight and the amount of amniotic fluid present. Until 20 to 24 weeks pregnancy, the measurements in the table will closely reflect those of your own. After 24 weeks, however, there is an increasing discrepancy between big and small fetuses, so the table will not necessarily closely reflect the measurements of your own. There is also a wide range in amniotic fluid volume throughout pregnancy; the volumes presented in the table are averages.

The large differences seen in the sizes of babies at birth come mostly in the second half of pregnancy, particularly the last few months. You can see from the chart that at 28 weeks an average weight is 1.1 kg but by the due date the average is more than three times this figure (3.4 kg). This shows how important these last three months are in determining the ultimate size of your baby. How big *you* are depends far more on other factors such as the tightness of your abdominal muscles (most women look smallest in their first pregnancy) and your own body build.

ORGAN FUNCTION

All fetal organs must function from early in pregnancy if normal development is to occur. The fetus whose movement is restricted (as can occur in the rare situation when there is no amniotic fluid) might not achieve normal muscle development. The fetus swallows amniotic fluid (see figure 1.5), which then passes into the stomach. This can often be seen on ultrasound. Similarly, kidneys produce urine, and with ultrasound this can be seen in the bladder from as early as 12 weeks. The fetus intermittently empties its bladder but rarely totally because it can nearly always be seen on ultrasound.

The fetus even practises breathing motions prior to birth. While its oxygen exchange is across the placenta, it does expand its chest intermittently, especially later in pregnancy. This aids lung development and prepares its chest muscles for breathing after birth.

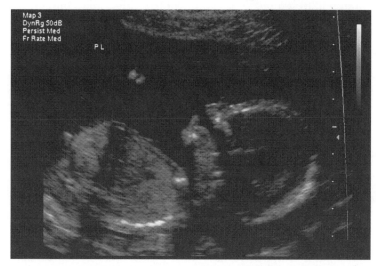

Figure 1.5 The fetus swallows the surrounding amniotic fluid. In this profile view, which shows the face up on the right, the mouth is open as the fetus swallows.

TABLE 1.2 MAIN STAGES IN FETAL DEVELOPMENT

WEEKS	DAYS	CROWN–RUMP LENGTH* (cm)	CROWN–HEEL LENGTH[†] (cm)	WEIGHT (gm)
0	0			
1	7			
2	14			
3	21			
4	28			
5	35			
6	42	0.3		
7	49	1		
8	56	1.6		
9	63	2.4		
10	70	3.3		

FEATURES PRESENT	APPEARANCE ON ULTRASOUND	VOLUME OF AMNIOTIC FLUID (ml)
First day of last menstrual period		
Ovulation (release of egg from ovary)		
Embryo implants in the wall of the uterus.		
Eyes and ears start to form, head and tail present.	Chorion becoming visible, pregnancy sac and embryo not seen.	
Arms start to form.	Pregnancy sac visible, but not embryo.	
Spinal canal closes around spinal cord.	Embryo and its heart movements visible.	1
Head and body well established.	Different structures of the embryo cannot yet be made out.	2
First movements occur. Chorion still totally surrounds pregnancy sac.	Head can be differentiated from body.	10
Fingers separated but toes still united. Chorion thicker where placenta will develop.	Arms and legs can be seen.	18
Heart fully formed, mature placenta. Now called a fetus. Human appearance with eyes, eyelids and ears.	Starts to look human with face, arms and legs seen.	34

TABLE 1.2 CONTINUED

WEEKS	DAYS	CROWN–RUMP LENGTH* (cm)	CROWN–HEEL LENGTH† (cm)	WEIGHT (gm)
11	77	4.3		
12	84	5.5		
13	91	6.8		
16			15	0.1
20			23	0.4
24			28	0.6
28			37	1.1
32			43	1.7
36			47	2.6
40			49	3.4

* Crown–rump length: the length from the top of the head to the tip of the bottom.
† Crown–heel length: the length from the top of the head to the heel when fetus is lying flat at its full length.

FEATURES PRESENT	APPEARANCE ON ULTRASOUND	VOLUME OF AMNIOTIC FLUID (ml)
Bowel returns inside fetal abdomen.	Spine, skull and some internal organs visible.	51
Urine production. Sex can be identified.		74
End of first 3 months (first trimester).	Improving views of fetal structure	110
Some pregnant women begin to feel movements	Usually can obtain good views of fetal organs.	200
Most pregnant women now feel movements.	'Screening' ultrasound performed 18–20 weeks.	
Babies delivered after this time have a chance of survival.	Good lifelike pictures of the fetus can still be seen.	
Eyelids open.	Fetus larger than transducer so couples find pictures harder to interpret.	1000
Babies delivered now unlikely to have severe complications of prematurity.	Most scans performed are to check fetal growth or the site of the placenta.	
Nails reach finger tips		
The due date (9 months + 7 days after the first day of last menstrual period)		600

The passageways to the lungs are full of fluid, which moves up and down with each 'breath'.

AMNIOTIC FLUID

Once the fetal kidneys start functioning at 8 to 9 weeks they soon produce most of the amniotic fluid. This is then removed by swallowing and is absorbed in the intestine. The whole volume of amniotic fluid is turned over at least once per day. The amount increases very rapidly in early pregnancy. At 6 weeks there is approximately 1 ml, by 10 weeks 34 ml and by 16 weeks 200 ml. As shown in table 1.2, the amount continues to increase slowly throughout the pregnancy until approximately 32 weeks and then decreases slightly until the due date.

There is a wide variation in the amount of fluid around fetuses at all stages of pregnancy. A little more or less than average in any particular pregnancy certainly does not suggest a problem. The fetus needs very little fluid around it to allow normal development. Only if the fluid is very much increased or decreased would your obstetrician be concerned. The worry is usually not the altered amount of fluid itself but rather what has *caused* this to happen (see chapter 2).

The content of the amniotic fluid tells us a great deal about the fetus, since it contains cells shed from the skin, lining of the airways, and other parts of the fetal body. Although most are dead, some are still alive and can be grown in the laboratory after the fluid has been sampled at amniocentesis. It is then possible to determine the chromosome count of the fetus or look for many other genetic diseases.

There is much more than just fetal cells floating in the amniotic fluid. Many sorts of protein, salts and hormones are found in it. The levels of many of these can be tested to study specific functions of the fetus. One example is alpha-fetoprotein (AFP), the level of which is raised in most instances of spina bifida. This will be discussed further in chapter 5. A further example is a test for bilirubin level in the amniotic fluid, which is used to assess the severity of blood group incompatibility in Rhesus disease. This will be discussed in chapter 11.

Questions

Is it going to be a big baby?

The answer to this question will not be evident if the scan is carried out in the first half of pregnancy. Even if it is going to be much larger or smaller than an average baby at birth, it is likely to be the same size as everybody else's until at least 20 weeks.

Is the pregnancy attached properly?

This concern is raised by women who have bleeding in early pregnancy. If the fetus is alive, then the pregnancy is properly attached. It attaches to the wall of the uterus 6 days after you conceive, so that by the time it is visible on the ultrasound screen it has been attached for some time.

Does the placenta look normal?

Placentas are remarkably consistent in appearance on ultrasound, and in early pregnancy the texture almost always appears the same. Occasionally towards the end of pregnancy the placenta might show some calcification and other changes, but even these do not mean there will be any problem with fetal growth or development. The important thing is the function of the placenta, and this is assessed by looking at the amount of amniotic fluid around the fetus, by the fetal growth, or by other tests.

chapter 2

Why have an Ultrasound Scan?

The number of ultrasound examinations that a pregnant woman should have is one of the most hotly debated topics in medicine today. This chapter discusses the reasons for women being offered 'routine' ultrasound scans, some of the arguments for and against this widespread practice, and the role of ultrasound in managing complications of pregnancy. It also examines some of the reasons why further scans might be suggested.

Ultrasound examinations use sound waves above the range of human hearing to provide images of the fetus. The advantages of being able to look at the fetus before birth has made the technique an almost universal part of safe obstetrics in Western countries. It is currently the safest and most non-invasive method of checking on fetal development. With the increasing sophistication of equipment, ultrasound has also become an invaluable method for diagnosing pregnancy complications and many fetal abnormalities.

ROUTINE ULTRASOUND

Increasingly doctors are offering all pregnant women an ultrasound examination at 18 to 20 weeks. The four main reasons are:

(i) **Dates**   It is impossible to be absolutely certain how far on a pregnancy is without an ultrasound examination. Confirmation or establishment by ultrasound of a due date simplifies the management of many obstetric complications.

(ii) **Multiple pregnancy**   Without ultrasound multiple pregnancies are usually diagnosed late in pregnancy, some twins only being detected after delivery of the first baby. This poses added risks to the babies.

(iii) **Placental localization**   A scan will pick out those who are at high risk of having a placenta which is too low in the uterus (placenta praevia). This can lead to bleeding late in pregnancy, in which case hospitalization is necessary.

(iv) **Malformations** Many malformations can now be detected by ultrasound. The range is so wide that these are covered separately in chapter 4 with a description of how they are visualized during the examination. Most babies with abnormalities are born to women who have had no previous problems. Therefore, if scans were restricted to those in high-risk groups, most abnormal fetuses would not be detected before birth.

There is also another factor that should not be forgotten. Couples often find their ultrasound examination an enjoyable and emotional experience. The pictures of the fetus obtained unquestionably help couples bond to their unborn child.

An ultrasound examination may be requested at other times for specific reasons:

(i) In the first three months (first trimester) ultrasound scans are not usually ordered routinely but are requested for complications, such as bleeding, or to determine dates. Since this is the most accurate time to determine dates a scan may be recommended if the due date is uncertain, particularly if an amniocentesis or CVS is planned, or so that the correct time to take blood for a serum screening test is known. For those seeking a no-risk test for Down syndrome, 10 to 13 weeks is the best time to look for indications on ultrasound scan (see chapter 8).

(ii) In the last three months of pregnancy (third trimester) ultrasound scans are not routine in most countries, but are carried out when there is concern about a specific issue, such as fetal growth.

(iii) In the second three months (second trimester) the most common time to have an ultrasound scan is at 18 to 20 weeks. This is now routinely offered in most Western countries. Several large studies have been published on routine ultrasound at 18 to 20 weeks, the largest of which is the RADIUS study, which received wide coverage in the international press. The RADIUS study authors concluded that there was no improvement in outcome for the pregnant woman or the fetus as a result of routine ultrasound examination. Their results, however, have been widely criticized. A low-risk, highly selected group of women was used in the study, and therefore the results cannot be extrapolated to any 'normal' population. Despite it being such a low-risk group, the obstetrician felt in necessary to order an ultrasound examination in nearly half of the women who should not have had a scan. Therefore, even if a scan is not done routinely, most women will end up having one anyway.

A number of benefits of routine ultrasound were shown in the RADIUS study, although only in the detection of abnormalities was there a statistical improvement in the outcome. Analysis of the study shows that if the ultrasound scan was performed by a highly skilled operator then not only was there an improved detection rate of abnormalities but there was also arguably a cost benefit involved in performing the scan. Another large study, this time from Finland, showed that routine ultrasound significantly reduced the number of perinatal deaths, that is, deaths late in pregnancy or immediately after birth.

Although the topic of routine scanning at 18 to 20 weeks is still being debated, the majority of obstetricians now believe that not only is there a benefit in offering all pregnant women an ultrasound scan but there is also a cost saving. In pregnant women who are sure of their last menstrual period (so the dates are relatively certain), the major reason for a routine ultrasound scan at 18–20 weeks is to check for fetal abnormality. Therefore, if the pregnant woman does not want a test for fetal abnormality, ultrasound is of limited benefit.

Women who have recently been on the oral contraceptive pill, or who are uncertain of dates, are recommended to have a scan to confirm the due date.

ARGUMENTS AGAINST ROUTINE ULTRASOUND

There are several disadvantages in every pregnant woman having an ultrasound examination. One is the financial cost, both to the individual and to the community. Another possible drawback is ill effects from the ultrasound itself. As discussed in chapter 3, it is now considered most unlikely that ultrasound used for diagnosis can cause damage to the fetus.

Another argument occasionally put against ultrasound is that it might lead to unnecessary intervention in the pregnancy. This could arise where there was an incorrect diagnosis of a problem, which led to inappropriate action. Such situations provide a strong argument for the use of good equipment and experienced operators, and if there is any doubt about a diagnosis, a second opinion; they do not constitute a valid argument against ultrasound itself.

TIMING OF THE SCAN

The appropriate timing for your ultrasound examination depends on the reason for having it. If it is undertaken because of bleeding, that dictates when it is carried out. If it is important that your dates be known exactly, then the scan should be done in the first few months of pregnancy. For most women, however, the best time to have a scan is at approximately 18 weeks. This is still quite a good time for checking the dates — to an accuracy of within one week — and multiple pregnancy and the placental site can readily be seen. At this time excellent views of the fetus can usually be obtained, which enables the detection of many abnormalities. Your obstetrician may have good reason for wanting to have the scan at a different time, but would discuss this with you.

CHECKING YOUR DATES

If the only thing that ultrasound could do was tell the age of a pregnancy it would still have a most important role to play in obstetrics. The management of complications is critically dependent on the age of the pregnancy. Before ultrasound, it was not possible for an obstetrician to be sure whether a small fetus in late pregnancy was the result of incorrect dates or inadequate growth. A number of women were confined to hospital, often for many weeks, in an effort to resolve this question. Widespread use of ultrasound has solved the problem because the age of any fetus can now be known precisely.

This also means of course that the exact time of conception can be known, which is important if the fetus might have been exposed to some potentially dangerous substance in early pregnancy. As women do not know they are pregnant until after they miss a period, and occasionally much later than this, they may unwittingly expose the fetus to various substances or medications. It then becomes important to know the date of conception to work out at what stage of fetal development the exposure occurred. Another reason for wanting to know the exact date is if there is doubt about the paternity (father's identity). Knowing the exact date of conception might help to tell who the father is.

No matter how sure you are of when you conceived, it is known that occasionally mistakes occur. Even though you know the date of your last period and even if you feel you know when you ovulated, nature can fool you. Occasionally what seems to be a 'last normal

menstrual period' was in fact bleeding in early pregnancy. If you conceived a month earlier and had some vaginal bleeding of an amount
and timing very similar to your period, then how would you know?
The surer you are of your cycle and conception date, the less likely it
is that such confusion will occur, but it still occasionally happens.
Also, many women do not ovulate exactly two weeks after the last
menstrual period, which complicates the calculation of the due date.

Similarly, a pelvic examination might not give a precise date. If,
for example, you have a fibroid or ovarian cyst, or even just a little
urine in your bladder, then the uterus can feel a lot bigger than it
really is. The examination is made through your own body tissues
so that if you are fatter or thinner than average, this might cause
confusion. Often there is no obvious reason why you feel big or small.
Moreover, when a clinical examination is done, the obstetrician feels
the overall size of the uterus, which includes the placenta and
amniotic fluid.

None of this discussion means that everybody *must* have an
ultrasound examination to work out how far on they are. If you are
sure when your last period began and your obstetrician feels that your
uterus is an appropriate size for these dates then there is only a low
chance that these clinical methods will prove to be inaccurate.

Don't forget that ultrasound does not tell you when you will
deliver your baby but rather when it is *due* to be delivered. You may
deliver well before the expected date or after it. There is no way, with
ultrasound or any other method, of predicting when your labour will
actually commence.

Timing of Scan for Checking Dates

The earlier the scan is performed, the more accurate is the due date
it will give you. This is because no matter what race the parents are,
how big they are, or how big the baby is destined to be at birth, its
growth rate is constant in the first few months. At 7 to 10 weeks
ultrasound will give a due date with an accuracy of a few days, and
this is therefore the best time for determining the date of conception.
Between 13 and 20 weeks the accuracy is to within one week either
way. The nearer you get to your due date, the less accurate it becomes.
In the second half of pregnancy there is a large biological variation in
growth rates, resulting in normal birth weights between about 2.9 kg
and 4.0 kg or more. Since with ultrasound the age of a pregnancy is
calculated by measuring parts of the fetus, clearly the method will be
very inaccurate in the last few weeks of pregnancy. In late pregnancy,

the date estimated by ultrasound may be as much as three or four weeks out.

Measurements for Determining Dates

Until 13 weeks the measurement taken is the 'crown–rump length' of the fetus (figure 1.3). This is a measurement taken from the top of the head to the tip of the bottom. If the fetus is too small for such details to be seen then the longest measurable length is taken to be the crown–rump length.

After 13 weeks any number of different measurements can be taken. Most people would measure three or even more parts of the fetus to help get the most accurate due date. The first used and probably still the most accurate measurement is that of the head — the biparietal diameter (BPD). The BPD is the largest measurement taken from one side of the skull to the other. While this can vary somewhat with the shape of the fetal head, it remains the most widely used measurement.

The second measurement is that of a long bone in one of the limbs, usually the femur (the bone of the thigh — see figure 4.11). The size of the fetal abdomen is usually also measured, particularly late in pregnancy. While the abdominal size is a most important measurement in assessing fetal growth (which we will look at later in this chapter) it can also be used to help determine how far on you are. Any number of other measurements can also be taken, but if the due dates provided by these first measurements correspond there is little to be gained.

MULTIPLE PREGNANCIES

Approximately one in 80 pregnancies conceived without the aid of medical treatment are twins, and one in 6400 are triplets. Ultrasound can identify the number of fetuses present from very early on in the pregnancy. No matter how early you are scanned, it is unlikely that ultrasound will miss twins. As a scan provides a section all the way through the pregnancy, the fetuses cannot 'hide behind one another' and avoid detection.

It is not until about 6 weeks that the fetuses and their heartbeats become visible in each of the pregnancy sacs. At this time, the number of fetuses seen is likely to be the number that you take home. If one dies, it will stay inside your uterus until the time of delivery, unlike a single pregnancy, which eventually miscarries after the death of the fetus. Its presence should not affect the growth and development of the other fetus. Without ultrasound, a pregnant woman would not be able to tell that a twin had died: the other fetus usually keeps growing normally, the placenta still operates, and there is no bleeding.

Identical Twins

Approximately 70 per cent of twins are non-identical (dizygous — coming from two separate eggs fertilized by two different sperm) and 30 per cent identical (monozygous — from one egg, which separates into two very early in development). Ultrasound can usually indicate whether the twins are likely to be identical. In the rare case where they are both in the same pregnancy sac without any membrane between, then they are always identical. If they are in sacs separated by a thin membrane, they are also likely to be identical. A thick membrane indicates a high chance of the twins being non-identical (figure 2.1). The presence of a single placenta, however, does *not* tell

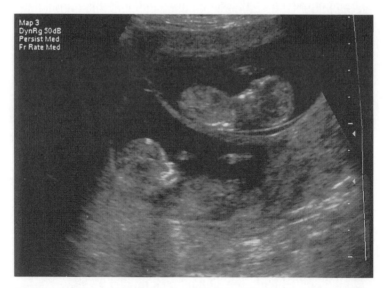

Figure 2.1 Twins at 10 weeks lying as if in bunk-beds, the top one with its head on the right, the bottom one with its head on the left — both faces looking upwards. The thick line that separates the fetuses indicates that the twins are dichorionic (implanted separately). Most dichorionic twins are non-identical.

you whether the twins will be identical. Approximately half of non-identical twins share a single placenta, although they each have their own circulation through separate parts of the placenta. Identical twins usually, however, have some mixing of their circulations at the placenta.

Siamese Twins

Siamese or conjoined twins are very rare — approximately one in 50 000 live births or one in 600 twin pregnancies. Nearly all twins are in their own separate sacs, which makes it impossible for them to be joined. Once the membrane between the fetuses has been identified then the possibility of joined twins can be immediately excluded.

Extra Scans

It is difficult for your obstetrician to feel each fetus individually through your abdominal wall if you have a multiple pregnancy. It may be suggested, therefore, that you have an ultrasound examination in the last few months of pregnancy to check the growth of each fetus. If it is difficult to feel which way the fetuses are lying, then this may be checked as well. There is no fixed time that such scans should be carried out.

PLACENTAL SITE

To understand what it means when the placenta appears to be low in early pregnancy requires an understanding of the development of the placenta. In the first 8 weeks of pregnancy the placenta, then called the chorion, surrounds all of the developing fetus and its pregnancy sac (figure 2.2). From 9 weeks, the placenta begins to thicken around one side of the pregnancy sac, and to thin around the rest of the pregnancy sac, to form the placenta. With the growth of the pregnancy the placenta occupies a smaller proportion of the wall of the uterus. By 18 weeks it occupies about one third of the wall of the uterus and by the time of birth about one sixth of the wall of the uterus. Not surprisingly, therefore, when a scan is carried out at 18 weeks the placenta will more often appear to be low lying than at the end of the pregnancy. While placenta praevia occurs only in about one in 200 pregnancies, the placenta looks low in up to one in 20 pregnancies at 18 weeks.

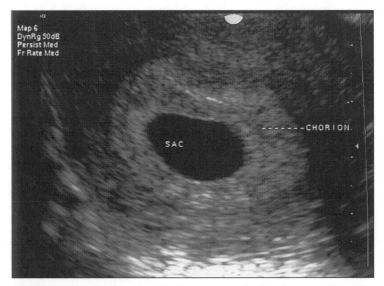

Figure 2.2 A blighted ovum. This pregnancy contained no fetus or yolk sac. The surrounding chorion is visible.

In around nine out of ten instances where the placenta appears to be low lying at around 18 weeks it will not be low lying at the time of delivery. Be carefully examining the exact position of the placenta, a skilled operator can estimate the chance of the placenta still being low at the time of delivery.

To be told that the placenta is low lying at 18 weeks therefore should not cause undue anxiety. There is usually no great concern from a medical viewpoint — it is simply an indication that a further scan should be carried out later in pregnancy to determine the ultimate position of the placenta. In the meantime there is no reason to alter your activities or lifestyle in any way, unless advised to do so by your obstetrician.

COMPLICATIONS IN PREGNANCY
Bleeding in Early Pregnancy

Bleeding in the first half of pregnancy is called a threatened abortion. If you are going to miscarry this is almost always the first sign you will have. About one in seven recognized pregnancies miscarry. In some pregnancies, however, women have bleeding even though the fetus is healthy and growing normally.

Ultrasound is the only test that will tell you whether the fetus is alive in early pregnancy. A pregnancy test only tells you that you are pregnant, and you probably already know that. Pregnancy tests merely tell you that there is some placental tissue present; they give little information about the well-being of the fetus itself.

Some obstetricians would always order an ultrasound examination if there is bleeding in early pregnancy. They would argue that if the fetus has died further bleeding is likely to continue until some action is taken, therefore the earlier the ultrasound examination is carried out, the better. Other obstetricians, on the other hand, might feel that if the uterus appears on examination to be an appropriate size for your dates and the bleeding has not been heavy there is a high chance that the fetus will remain healthy and that it would be a waste of time and resources to perform a scan. Neither viewpoint will be correct in every case. Ultrasound does provide a good indication of whether you will miscarry. If the fetus is alive, with its heartbeat visible, there is approximately an 85 per cent chance that it will continue to develop normally.

It is worth noting that if bleeding occurs either the fetus has already died and you will miscarry, or it will continue to develop with little increased chance of having an abnormality. The blood that is lost is your own and not fetal. The placenta has great powers of recovery, so even if there is clot in the uterus it does not cause any damage to fetal health or growth.

Miscarriage

It might surprise you to know that, if you miscarry, the fetus has nearly always died some weeks or months before, usually in the first 8 weeks of pregnancy. The miscarriage itself may occur as late as 20 weeks. In the meantime you still feel pregnant, as the placenta continues to function and produce pregnancy hormones. You may even feel that you are still growing.

If your obstetrician does an internal examination, he or she may notice that your uterus feels a little smaller than it should, but otherwise there is no way of telling that the fetus has died. The symptoms you notice in early pregnancy, such as nausea, start to lessen after the death of the fetus, but these are often improving at this time anyway so are difficult to interpret. Don't be surprised and disappointed in your obstetrician if you have a miscarriage and find on the scan that the fetus has been dead for some time and nobody has suspected it.

If the fetus grows for at least the first 6 weeks and then fails to develop it can usually be seen on ultrasound and is called a 'missed abortion'. This is not 'missed' because it is lost but rather because it has died and your body has not yet expelled it (i.e. there has been no miscarriage). If, on the other hand, the fetus died earlier than this then it will be too small to be seen on ultrasound, and it is called a 'blighted ovum' (i.e. a pregnancy without a visible fetus — see figure 2.2). In either case, if nothing is done after the fetus has died then you will ultimately miscarry. As this may take many weeks or months, and may be associated with heavy blood loss, most women and their obstetricians believe that it is much better and safer to curette the uterus. Either situation will have no bearing on future pregnancies — after one miscarriage, the risk of a miscarriage in the next pregnancy is not increased.

If your pregnancy is 6 weeks or less when you have the scan performed, the fetal heartbeat cannot yet be seen. It is of course impossible to know whether it cannot be seen because it is too early or because the fetus is dead. Even if you believe you are further on than the size of the pregnancy suggests, it is hard to be certain, so it is best to repeat the scan one week later. Depending on the experience of your doctor and whether or not he or she has a vaginal scanner, it is sometimes even much later than this before you can be given a definite answer on ultrasound.

If the fetus is alive, the main features your doctor will look for which might indicate whether you are likely to miscarry subsequently are:

(i) If fetus is growing normally, but the amount of fluid around it in the pregnancy sac is very much reduced, then there is a much higher chance of later miscarriage. If the pregnancy continues the volume will slowly increase over the next few weeks with no harm occurring to the fetus.

(ii) On the scan it is occasionally also possible to see some blood clot, which would indicate where the bleeding has come from. If the amount of blood is small it has no influence on the developing fetus. If there is a large amount of blood clot present, however, there is an increased chance that you will miscarry subsequently. If a clot is visible in your uterus you might later lose a small amount of old brown blood from your vagina. Most of it will absorb from within the uterus, however, just as a bruise absorbs elsewhere in the body.

(iii) Rarely, the fetal heartbeat or growth rate is too slow.

Occasionally other features about the pregnancy might be noted on the scan report, such as where the placenta is developing, but in early pregnancy these do not appear to be of much consequence.

Causes of Miscarriage

While this topic is really outside the scope of this book, your obstetrician will tell you that we rarely discover why a fetus died. It is known that many or even most fetuses that die in early pregnancy do so because they had an abnormality, particularly of the chromosomes. The chance of it happening again in general is low. Many people wish to know the sex of the fetus they have lost, but, as the death usually occurs very early in the pregnancy, the sex cannot be seen on ultrasound. For your own peace of mind you should recognize that it did not die because of anything you did; you could not have prevented it happening. Although miscarriage is common, most couples find it extremely upsetting and experience similar feelings to couples who lose a child after birth.

Pain in Early Pregnancy

Pain in pregnancy can be persistent and worrying. It is important to realize that pain is rarely the first sign of a miscarriage. The first sign is bleeding, and if pain occurs it is later, when the bleeding becomes heavy and the uterus contracts.

Pain in pregnancy unassociated with bleeding is very common but usually has no serious underlying cause. However, three important conditions that can cause pelvic pain early on must be considered: ectopic pregnancy, ovarian cysts, and fibroids. Even when you have had no symptoms, these conditions may occasionally be suspected when your doctor feels a lump other than the pregnant uterus in the pelvis.

Ectopic pregnancy

An **ectopic pregnancy** is one that develops outside the uterine cavity, the commonest type being inside the fallopian tube (figure 2.3). This can be a serious, even life-threatening, ordeal, as an ectopic pregnancy tends to rupture and bleed internally. While occasionally there are reports of a pregnancy in the abdomen resulting in a healthy baby, this is extraordinarily rare. Because of the dangers, surgery is undertaken as soon as the diagnosis is suspected.

An ectopic pregnancy may be suspected by your doctor if you develop pain in early pregnancy or because you are at special risk

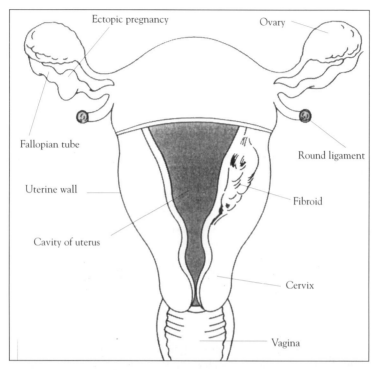

Figure 2.3 This diagram illustrates a non-pregnant uterus with the ovaries, fallopian tubes and round ligaments on each side. A fibroid is shown in the wall of the uterus. An ectopic pregnancy is illustrated in one tube.

— perhaps you have had a previous ectopic pregnancy, pelvic infection, an operation on the fallopian tubes, or infertility. This used to be a most difficult diagnosis for your doctor to make, but with ultrasound it is much easier.

There are two ways of making this diagnosis with ultrasound. If the ultrasound is performed using a vaginal scanner, the ectopic pregnancy can usually be seen outside the uterus. If the scan is done through the abdomen, such a pregnancy will not usually be visible. In this case, the diagnosis is made when a woman known to be pregnant has no visible pregnancy inside the uterus. Such women will often need to have surgery to confirm the diagnosis, usually a laparoscopy — an examination of the inside of the abdomen with a medical telescope.

It is important to realize that ultrasound cannot *exclude* the possibility of an ectopic pregnancy. If a healthy pregnancy is inside the uterus you could also have an ectopic pregnancy, although this is extraordinarily rare. Alternatively, no matter how good the scanning equipment and the operator, a small ectopic pregnancy could be present but not picked up on the scan. With modern equipment, however, this is happening less often.

Ovarian cysts
Every woman in early pregnancy has an **ovarian cyst**, known as the corpus luteum, which forms in the ovary after the release of the egg. Thin-walled, the cyst is full of fluid or blood and produces the hormones responsible for maintaining the pregnancy. It is generally small, between one and three centimetres in diameter, although occasionally it reaches five centimetres or more. The fluid in the cyst is usually absorbed over the first few months of pregnancy until it disappears totally. If there is a large cyst that persists after the first three months, an operation may be needed to remove it.

Occasionally ovarian cysts arise from other causes. On ultrasound, it is often possible to differentiate them from a corpus luteum. They may be larger, usually five centimetres in diameter or more, and often contain septa (or partitions) inside the fluid. They may also contain solid tissue instead of fluid. Most of these are not cancerous — it is very rare indeed to have an ovarian cancer in pregnancy. Despite this, it would usually be recommended that cysts containing solid areas be removed at around 14 weeks, or earlier if they are associated with severe pain.

Fibroids
Fibroids, or fibromyomata, to use their proper name, are thickenings of muscle and fibrous tissue in the wall of the uterus. They are very common, particularly in women over 40 years old (figure 2.3). They can reach a very large size, but they virtually never become cancerous. It is also very rare for them to interfere with the development or health of the fetus. The main problems they present are, first, that they may be difficult to diagnose and can be confused with an ovarian cyst, although usually they can be differentiated on ultrasound; second, they may be a source of pain in pregnancy. This may be of the greatest nuisance to you but still does not interfere with fetal development. They are virtually never removed in pregnancy because the muscle of the uterus has such a rich blood supply that it

would be difficult to control the bleeding. Very occasionally a fibroid low in the uterus may obstruct the birth of the baby.

Other Causes of Pain

If you have pain and ultrasound shows a healthy pregnancy and no cyst or fibroid, then what is the cause? It may be due to a problem in your bowel or elsewhere but these are rarely detectable with ultrasound. If no cause is found then it is usually considered to be 'round ligament pain', due to stretching of the round ligament that helps support the uterus (see figure 2.3). If this is the cause of your pain then no abnormality is seen on ultrasound. The pain can be a nuisance over a moderately long period of the pregnancy, but it does ultimately settle down, usually in the middle stages. It causes no disturbance to the growth or well-being of the fetus so you need have no fears.

Bleeding in Late Pregnancy

The causes of bleeding in the second half of pregnancy are different from those in the first half. When bleeding occurs in the second half, the concern is the location of the placenta. Bleeding after 20 weeks may be due to the placenta being too low in your uterus, a condition known as placenta praevia (figure 2.4). If this happens the bleeding

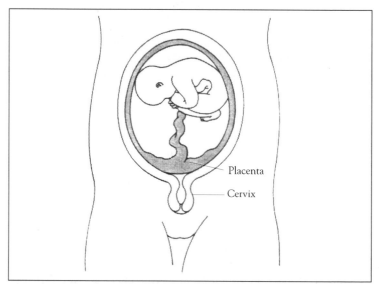

Figure 2.4 Placenta praevia: The placenta lies over the inside of the cervix.

is likely to recur, so you may have to remain in hospital and have the baby delivered by Caesarean section. Ultrasound is very accurate at diagnosing a low-lying placenta. It is, however, less accurate in diagnosing the other major cause of bleeding after 20 weeks, namely accidental haemorrhage. This is bleeding behind a normally sited placenta, which, if not severe or persistent, should not require prolonged hospitalization.

OTHER THINGS ULTRASOUND CAN TELL YOU
Sex of the Fetus

'Can you tell the sex?' is a very common question pregnant women ask their ultrasound operator. At first you may think this question is the same as 'Please tell me the sex'. It is not. Most pregnant women wish to know if the doctor can tell the sex, but only some actually wish to know themselves. The decision whether to find out the sex of the unborn baby is of critical importance to many couples. Commonly one wishes to know and the other does not. The one who decides against knowing may or may not be happy for his or her partner to know. Many pregnant women appear determined to find out the sex of the fetus, but when told that the sex cannot be seen are relieved. In addition, some obstetricians are happy for all their patients to find out the sex while others feel that this is not a good idea. In the middle of all these strong emotions sits the doctor performing the scan wondering what to do. If you and your partner do wish to know the sex, make this clear at the start of the scan.

There is no truth in the widely held belief that the fetal heart rate indicates the sex. To determine the sex of a fetus, the doctor looks at the genitals as shown in figures 2.5 and 2.6. The middle stage of pregnancy is the best time; by 18 weeks the sex of most fetuses can be seen, but prior to 13 weeks it can be difficult. Towards the end of pregnancy, when there is less amniotic fluid around the fetus in relation to it's size, it may again be hard to tell the sex. If the fetal back is uppermost (i.e. the fetus is facing your spine), it is usually impossible to be sure.

Do not count on the sex of the fetus when seen on ultrasound as an absolute guarantee. It should, however, have an accuracy rate in the order of 98 per cent, depending on the stage of pregnancy, the experience of the doctor, and the position of the fetus. Ask how confident the doctor is about the sex.

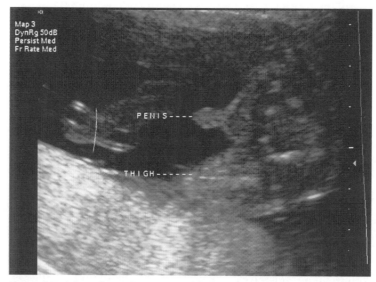

Figure 2.5 A boy: the penis and scrotum are visible (a section of cord is floating in front of the penis).

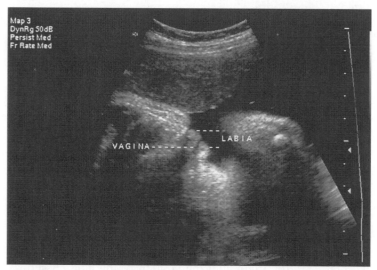

Figure 2.6 A girl: the labia are visible on either side of the vagina.

Occasionally couples ask to have the sex determined early on so they can have the pregnancy terminated if it is not what they want. Most doctors feel that this is an inappropriate use of powerful technology, and, by the time the doctor can be certain of the sex, the fetus is likely to be too advanced for an abortion to be readily performed. In any case, most doctors would have difficulty accepting the sex of the fetus as a legitimate ground for abortion, as it is a precedent for 'positive eugenics'.

Fetal Growth

One of the main aims of obstetric care is to monitor fetal growth. Your obstetrician would very much like to be able to calculate the weight exactly. How well the fetus grows depends on the adequacy of the nutrition it receives across the placenta. If this is inadequate then there is an increased risk of a number of complications, including being stillborn. Growth assessment is usually done by your obstetrician palpating your abdomen, but if there are doubts about the growth an ultrasound examination may be ordered.

The aim of an ultrasound in this instance is to 'weigh' the fetus. Clearly this is not possible before birth. Instead, two or three measurements are taken, particularly those of the abdomen, head and femur. The approximate current weight is calculated from these measurements using charts. It cannot be precise, as the fetal body build, such as the amount of fat around their arms and legs, varies. It is, however, the best method available and will give a weight estimate to within 10 per cent accuracy approximately 75 per cent of the time. It will not, of course, tell you what its weight will be at birth. Nobody can tell when you will deliver and what the growth will be like in the intervening period.

Using ultrasound, there are features other than fetal growth that can be assessed to determine its nutritional status. These include the amount of both the amniotic fluid present and fatty tissue it is laying down. As discussed in chapter 1, looking at the placenta for signs of 'ageing' is not very helpful.

The purpose of monitoring fetal growth is to determine the optimal timing of delivery — to balance the risks of delivering it prematurely against those of leaving it undelivered. Only if fetal growth is severely reduced would your obstetrician start to wonder whether there could be an underlying genetic problem. Other tests may then be considered, such as sampling the baby's blood for a chromosomal abnormality (which will be discussed in chapter 11).

Fetal well-being

One of the greatest challenges in obstetrics is to find a test that will show if the well-being of the fetus is suddenly jeopardized. Its growth may be measured on ultrasound every two weeks to check on nutrition, but what if its condition deteriorated rapidly? There are a number of tests available, none of which provides the whole answer. The most common use different sorts of ultrasound equipment, so we will look at them briefly.

(i)   **Cardiotocography** (CTG) is the most widely used test, providing a tracing of the fetal heartbeat for some 20 to 40 minutes. Specific clearly defined variations in the heartbeat may indicate that the fetus is in jeopardy.

(ii) A **biophysical profile** provides a score to assess fetal well-being. The movements of the limbs, the 'breathing' movements and the amount of amniotic fluid around the fetus are examined with ultrasound, and a CTG may also be performed. Not widely used in Australia, this test is popular in North America and some other places. Fetuses that are in sudden distress tend to show no movements and there is usually a reduction in the amount of amniotic fluid around them.

(iii) **Fetal Doppler studies** are used as a test of well-being of the fetus in the middle and later stages of pregnancy. They involve the use of ultrasound equipment to check the patterns of blood flow through the blood vessels of the umbilical cord (figure 2.7). These patterns change if placental function is reduced.

Variations in the Amount of Amniotic Fluid

The amount of amniotic fluid around the fetus may vary widely in normal situations. The reason for a little more or less than average is usually not known and is of no consequence. Occasionally, however, the amount of fluid is either much greater than or less than what is accepted as normal.

If there is an excess of fluid around the fetus often no cause can be found, but it is likely to cause the pregnant woman increased discomfort. Occasionally it may be associated with a multiple pregnancy or a fetal abnormality. Amniotic fluid is largely removed by the fetus swallowing, so anything that prevents this, such as a blockage in the upper part of its intestine, can cause a fluid increase. Other causes include spina bifida, or a deficiency in the abdominal wall of the fetus through which its intestines protrude (called exomphalos). Most of these abnormalities can be seen on ultrasound, so if the fetus appears normal on a scan, the likelihood is that there is no

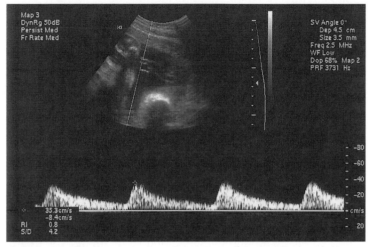

Figure 2.7 A Doppler examination of the artery of the umbilical cord. The top image shows a length of cord, and the two short parallel horizontal lines overlying it indicate that the sample is from within the cord. The pulsations in the cord's artery are visible in the bottom image.

abnormality causing the increase. If there is a very large amount of fluid, your obstetrician might consider further testing such as fetal blood sampling or placental biopsy to exclude a chromosomal abnormality.

A reduction in the amount of fluid around the fetus may be due to poor placental function. Your obstetrician would take extra care to watch fetal growth. Occasionally there is no or minimal fluid around a fetus. This may result from the fetus not passing urine into the amniotic fluid due to inadequate or blocked kidney function or because of a severe reduction in blood flow through the placenta. (It might also be because your waters have broken but in this case you would usually be aware of fluid draining from the vagina.) A severe reduction in the amount of amniotic fluid may also be an indication for further testing of the fetus.

ULTRASOUND DOES NOT GUARANTEE A NORMAL BABY

Ultrasound is no panacea. Like any other test undertaken on the fetus, it does not guarantee it will be normal. We all know a child may look totally normal and yet have some severe problems, such as intellectual disability. Ultrasound is just a method of looking at a fetus, albeit a more sophisticated method than merely looking at the features of a child after birth with the naked eye. With ultrasound we can see not only the parts of the body visible after birth, like arms, legs and face, but also many of the internal organs. It is an excellent method for examining the structure of many of these organs but usually not their function. It can show in beautiful detail the structure of the brain but it will tell you nothing of how well that brain works. If there is intellectual impairment due to hydrocephaly (water on the brain) this will be seen on ultrasound, but unfortunately most intellectually disabled babies have normal brain structure.

Remember that ultrasound can only detect abnormalities present at the time of the scan. Occasionally, abnormalities develop late in pregnancy, although most are present from a very early stage. Ultrasound is also not a good way of looking at adult bones. It cannot therefore tell if your pelvic size will be adequate for delivery.

Questions

Where has the bleeding come from?

This is often asked in relation to bleeding in early pregnancy. If a scan shows a blood clot in the uterus, outside but adjacent to the pregnancy sac, then this is where the bleeding has arisen. In the absence of such a clot it is impossible to know the source of bleeding, but it is usually presumed to be somewhere adjacent to the developing placenta.

Will the bleeding damage the unborn baby?

No. Bleeding in early pregnancy causes few if any long-term problems. If you do not miscarry, the fetus should continue to develop normally.

When did the fetus die?

This is commonly asked when a fetus has died in early pregnancy. The crown–rump length of the fetus gives a good indication of how advanced it was when it died. Couples like to work out what they were doing at the time of death to see what could have caused it. This is a fruitless task as the cause is almost always unknown and often some innocuous event or activity is inappropriately blamed.

I know when I conceived, so why does the scan give a different date?

The first source of confusion is that obstetricians, for convenience, take the beginning of pregnancy from the first day of the last period. If a woman feels she knows when she conceived she takes this date as the beginning of pregnancy. A conversation with your doctor can usually resolve this difference.

If you are certain of your dates and a scan done in the first half of pregnancy differs from this date by more than a week then the scan is nearly always correct.

Are the dates still correct?

Couples often ask this after a second or subsequent scan. The earlier in pregnancy a scan is done the more accurate it is at predicting a due date. It would be inappropriate to change the date as a result of a scan done later in the pregnancy. A second scan is good at telling how the fetus is growing but less precise at predicting a due date.

When will my baby be born?

Ultrasound can give a very accurate due date, but of course nobody can tell if the baby will be born on that day. Some babies come very early and some very late. This unpredictable timing of the onset of labour is one of the mysteries of pregnancy.

Are my twins joined?

In a multiple pregnancy each fetus nearly always has its own separate bag of waters. If the membrane between the fetuses can be seen, and it nearly always can, this means that the fetuses could not be joined.

Are the twins identical?

The best way of working this out is by looking at the placenta and the membrane between the fetuses. If there are two placentas or the membrane is thick they are probably not identical. It should be noted that single placenta is common with identical twins, but also with non-identical twins.

What is a low-lying placenta?

Early in pregnancy the placenta totally surrounds the pregnancy sac. By the end of the pregnancy the placenta occupies only a small portion of the wall of the uterus. The placenta in early pregnancy therefore often looks low but becomes normally sited later on. It takes experience to know how low a normal placenta can be at any particular stage of pregnancy. If there is any doubt, a second scan may be performed late in pregnancy to eliminate the possibility of placenta praevia.

Will we know the sex of the fetus?

It takes experience to tell the sex and unless it is specifically pointed out you will not be able to see it. If you wish to know the sex, it is a good idea to mention this in advance. The genitals of the fetus need to be closely examined to be sure of the sex, and usually the doctor will not do this unless specifically requested. It is sometimes possible to see the sex as early as 13 weeks and usually possible by 16 to 20 weeks.

Can you see how fast the fetal heart is beating?

Yes, you can always count the heartbeat. It is, however, very rarely of any consequence. Except in extreme circumstances, it does not indicate how healthy the fetus is. It does not even tell you what the sex is, despite many an old wives' tale.

Is the size of my pelvis normal?

Ultrasound provides poor pictures of adult bones and is unable to tell you this.

Is the position of the fetus causing my pain?

In the first half of pregnancy lower abdominal pains are common. Pregnant women often blame the way the fetus is lying, but this is an unlikely cause. Such pains may be due to a fibroid (a thickening of muscle and fibrous tissue in the wall of the uterus) or a cyst on the ovary. If neither of these is seen on ultrasound, the pain is often said to be caused by ligaments stretching. It produces no ill effects on the fetus and will usually settle in midpregnancy.

My ultrasound suggests the pregnancy is less advanced than I expected. Could it be that the fetus is not growing normally?

It is very rare for there to be significant alterations in growth of a fetus in the first half of pregnancy. If there is poor growth, other signs, such as a reduced amount of amniotic fluid, are usually obvious. Hence, if the fetus is significantly larger or smaller than expected prior to 20 weeks it is nearly always because you did not conceive at exactly the time you calculated.

How long is the fetus?

As fetuses are curled up in the uterus, the 'stretched out' length cannot be measured. Ultrasound will be used mostly to detect diameters or bone lengths. The length of fetuses throughout pregnancy are shown in chapter 1.

Is the fetus lying the correct way?

Until the last three months of pregnancy the fetal position varies. While its position is readily seen using ultrasound, a few minutes later it may change and this is quite normal. Most fetuses will remain head first from 34 weeks or earlier.

Why does the fetal head look bigger than the body?

The diameter of the head exceeds that of the body throughout pregnancy until around 32 weeks. After 32 weeks fat starts to be deposited around the abdomen, which then becomes larger than the head.

chapter 3

The Ultrasound Examination

To get the most out of an ultrasound examination you need to know something about how it works and whether the procedure carries any risks. This chapter will look at how ultrasound works and provide a step-by-step account of the examination. There is a great variety of ultrasound equipment in use. Many units are adequate for simple examinations, but not sufficiently sophisticated to allow diagnosis of most abnormalities. This chapter aims to show you different types of equipment and what each can do.

WHAT IS ULTRASOUND?

A possible source of confusion is the many names used for the same test. As well as being called an ultrasound examination it is often referred to as a 'sonar' or 'scan' and may also be called an 'ultrasound scan', 'real-time scan', or 'sonar scan'. *Scan* is really a loose term for any test that provides pictures of the inside of your body. In fact, methods other than ultrasound are rarely used for looking at a fetus during pregnancy. Other imaging techniques provide less information in most situations.

Ultrasound examinations use sound waves similar to those in our speech. Dog whistles use a frequency above the range of human hearing; ultrasound is a far higher frequency still. Humans can hear frequencies between about one and 20 000 cycles per second, while ultrasound is usually one to 20 million cycles per second.

Sound waves we can hear travel readily in all directions through air. Ultrasound, however, has different properties. It does not travel through air, hence unless the transmitter actually touches you, no ultrasound reaches you. People watching the scan are therefore not exposed to any ultrasound.

Ultrasound also tends to travel in a straight line and, as shown in figure 3.1, can be made into a narrow beam like a torch light. Both

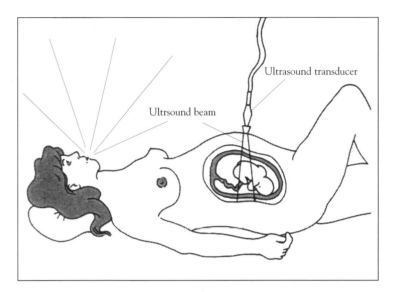

Figure 3.1   When we speak the sound waves travel through air in all directions whereas ultrasound uses sound waves, which travel through tissue but not air, and focus into a narrow beam like a beam of light.

the sound waves we hear and ultrasound have one important property in common — echoes occur when they hit an obstacle. Audible sound waves echo off a nearby wall or mountain, as shown in figure 3.2. Similarly, as ultrasound passes through the body, echoes bounce off each tissue layer. These echoes are registered by the machine to produce a picture.

HOW ULTRASOUND BEGAN

Ultrasound has been around longer than most people imagine, its medical use following development of the technology for other purposes. The Allies first developed sonar during the First World War for the detection of submarines. Industrial applications, such as flaw detection in metals, followed. In 1948, the first primitive pictures of a fetus were produced, heralding ultrasound's entry into medicine. By the end of the 1950s it had been used for diagnosis of conditions in many parts of the body.

It was in obstetrics and gynaecology that ultrasound made the greatest early impact. Professor Ian Donald from Glasgow is

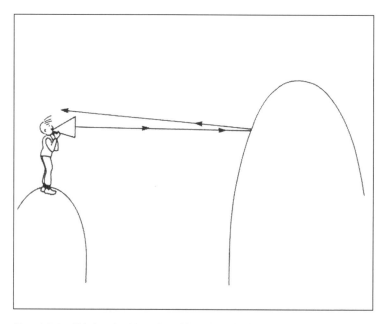

Figure 3.2 This boy is able to hear his voice echo from a distant mountain. In a similar way, ultrasound pictures are produced by transmitting sound waves through tissue which then echo back and are received, processed and displayed on a television screen.

acknowledged as the person who introduced ultrasound into clinical obstetrics in 1958. The first commercial ultrasound machine was available in 1963 and its use became widespread by the early 1970s. The beautifully detailed pictures we see today are a result of technological refinements made in the 1980s and 1990s.

ITS USE IN MEDICINE

Ultrasound may be used to treat conditions as well as to diagnose them. It is widely used at much higher power levels than in obstetrics to speed the healing of injuries and even to break up kidney stones. It is also commonly used to diagnose conditions throughout the body in people of all ages. In this book we will concentrate on its use in pregnancy.

Different types of ultrasound equipment are used in pregnancy. You may be surprised to learn that the 'microphone' used by obstetricians to listen to the fetal heartbeat when it cannot be heard by the stethoscope also uses ultrasound. Similarly, ultrasound equipment can trace the heartbeat of the fetus or be used to look at its blood flow when you are near the end of pregnancy.

HOW THE ULTRASOUND MACHINE WORKS

This section can be skipped by those people who are not interested in how the ultrasound equipment operates.

If we were to run an electric current across a crystal (transducer) of a material like quartz or a ceramic substance, the energy would be converted into sound waves. These can be 'beamed' in a specific direction through a patient's skin. As they traverse the body, they encounter various tissue interfaces from which they will be reflected back to the same transducer. This transducer then becomes a receiver and the sound waves are converted back into electric pulses. The machine takes the electrical information provided by the echoes and transforms it into a two-dimensional picture on a television monitor.

The pulses of sound are short, about a millionth of a second. They are fired about a thousand times per second. We can therefore already see one of the safety factors in the equipment — if the ultrasound machine is applied for one second, sound waves are only being applied for one thousandth of a second. The rest of the time is spent receiving the echoes between pulses. So if your examination takes thirty minutes (1800 seconds), then the ultrasound is only actively working for 1.8 seconds.

One of the great advances in the 1980s was the development of 'real-time' ultrasound equipment. 'Real-time' means that moving pictures of the fetus are produced instead of the old still ones. There are many ways that these moving pictures can be produced, and the methods are not important here, but they have one thing in common — they produce images of sections, or slices, of tissue (figure 3.3).

If the section is taken up and down a pregnant woman's abdomen, the inside of her abdomen in the long axis of her body is shown on the screen. In figure 3.3, the fetus is lying bottom down along the long axis of the pregnant woman so a section up and down her abdomen would show the whole length of the fetus. As it is a slice, all of the fetus is never on the same picture — if the head and body are on the screen, the limbs will usually not be visible. In

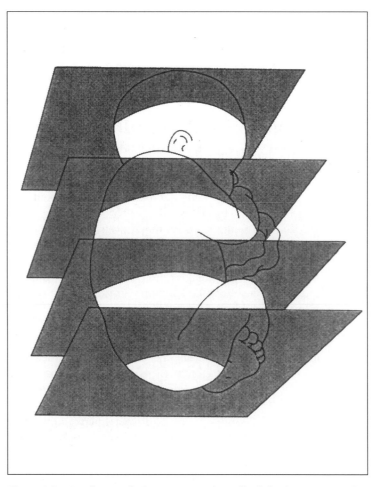

Figure 3.3 An ultrasound picture cannot show all of the fetus at once, but shows one section (or slice) through one part of the fetus at a time, similar to one of the sections shown here.

addition, since it is a slice, the insides of the fetus are visible, allowing its heart and other internal organs to be seen on the screen. It is like slicing a loaf of bread and examining each slice in turn. The operator can magnify part of the fetus so that none of the pregnant woman's tissues are visible on the screen.

As well as enabling us to *see* tissues, ultrasound makes it possible to take very accurate measurements. It is known that ultrasound travels through tissues at approximately 1540 metres per second. The machine measures how long it takes for sound waves to travel to a point, such as the fetal leg, and back. It can be designed to read out how far that leg is from the transducer since distance = time (which the machine knows) X speed of ultrasound (1540 metres per second)

Modern ultrasound machines use electronic calipers, which the operator freely moves around the television monitor to allow the distance between any two points to be accurately measured.

Although ultrasound pictures are usually only in black and white, colour ultrasound has an increasing place. Colour is used to show blood flow. In pregnancy colour is commonly used to look at the heart and at the blood vessels in the umbilical cord of the fetus. The red and blue colours show the direction of flow to and away from the ultrasound transducer respectively (many people wrongly think that the colours are red for arterial blood and blue for venous blood). Increasingly, colour ultrasound is being used to check the blood flow in the fetal heart in every pregnancy, but this is not yet routine.

Another development, which has been researched for many years, is the three-dimensional ultrasound machine, but these are not yet in widespread use. Three-dimensional ultrasound images may be the way of the future, but the current state of the technology means that they have few, if any, advantages.

THE EQUIPMENT

Anybody who had an ultrasound examination more than 10 years ago and then another one since could not help but notice that the equipment has been reduced in size. Early equipment used to fill half a moderate-sized room while the modern version (figure 3.4) is a relatively small unit sitting beside the couch. At the same time, there has been an increase in the range of transducers and a great improvement in the quality (or resolution) of the images. Ultrasound machines are now large computers with sophisticated software. Meanwhile, the price has unfortunately also increased, with some equipment now costing several times as much as the average house. Such equipment may only be available in regional centres and at specialist practices.

Small, cheaper equipment is widely available and is useful for basic work such as detecting twins and measuring the head size to calculate dates. To make the large number of more difficult diagnoses

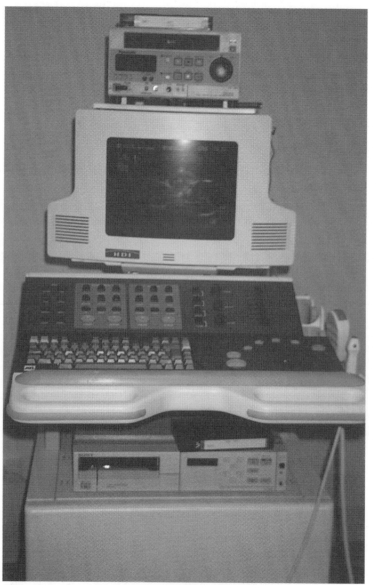

Figure 3.4 A current-generation ultrasound machine.

that are possible with ultrasound requires sophisticated (and expensive) state-of-the-art equipment. You may find it difficult to recognize such equipment; one way of assessing the level of sophistication of the kind used by your doctor would be to ask if it was good for diagnosing such structural abnormalities as heart abnormalities.

WHO SHOULD PERFORM THE SCAN?

As important as the quality of the equipment is the expertise of the operator. When you have your ultrasound examination you will want to know that it is being performed by an expert. As a rule of thumb, if the aim of the scan is to check the fetus thoroughly for abnormalities, more than 750 examinations a year should be undertaken to maintain experience. The scan may be carried out by your own doctor, by a specialist in ultrasound, or by a technician known as a sonographer. In the latter case, the pictures are later interpreted and reported by the doctor. All methods can work well with appropriately trained and experienced personnel. Many ultrasound courses and examinations are available. For some of the more simple examinations, such as checking the heartbeat or the position of the fetus, fewer examinations are needed to maintain expertise. Experience in looking at fetuses is at least as important as the qualifications a person holds.

CAN ULTRASOUND DAMAGE THE FETUS?

Hundreds of scientific reports on the safety of ultrasound have been published and none has found any reproducible ill effects. The Australiasian Society for Ultrasound in Medicine, whose brief is to watch the scientific literature continuously, published a statement in May 1993 regarding grey-scale (black and white) imaging, from which the following is extracted:

> To date the results of numerous follow-up studies on patients and children who had been examined before birth have failed to demonstrate any significant biological effects that could be attributed to this mode of examination . . .

Given the known benefits and efficacy of the medical diagnosis, the prudent use of grey-scale imaging far outweighs the risks, if any, that may be present. There is no reason to withhold the application of the technique when it is indicated on clinical grounds.

Similar statements have been produced by equivalent organizations in other countries.

Research into the effects of ultrasound includes laboratory studies of cell changes, animal research, and follow-up studies of babies exposed to ultrasound. In each case no reproducible ill effects have been shown to result. A well-designed study reported in 1984 involved 425 babies who underwent ultrasound examination prior to birth and 381 matched controls, babies of similar background who were not scanned. Physical development and tests of nerve function were compared at birth and again between 7 and 12 years, revealing no significant differences.

One of the most widely publicized adverse reports was of changes in the chromosomes of cells exposed to ultrasound. This report has not been confirmed by other workers using the same methods, so it is believed that the reported chromosome changes must have been caused by some other agent. Another recent study has suggested that babies born after frequent ultrasound examinations tend to be slightly smaller than those not exposed to ultrasound. It is unclear whether this difference in size was directly related to ultrasound or whether it could have been caused by some other factors, so further study is required. The difference in size was very small (an average of only 30 grams per baby) and could no longer be detected at one year, and there was no suggestion that the babies involved suffered any adverse consequences. While there has been criticism of some studies investigating possible harmful effects of ultrasound, the sheer number showing no ill effect has reassured physicists, obstetricians and radiologists that ultrasound examinations are safe. Confidence in its safety has reached such a level that it has become a routine procedure in pregnancy in many countries. Indeed, in Germany the law demands that every pregnant woman must be offered two ultrasound examinations by her doctor, one early in pregnancy and one late, and many have a scan at every antenatal visit.

There are several factors that reduce the possibility of harm from ultrasound. When examining a pregnancy, low power levels are used. In the previous section we explained that ultrasound uses extremely short pulses of sound, so that the transducer is only sending out sound waves for approximately one thousandth of the examination time.

Also, only part of the fetus is seen on the screen at one time, so the rest of it is receiving minimal ultrasound exposure. Thus any one part of the fetus receives ultrasound for a very short time during the examination.

It has been known for a long time that ultrasound at much higher power levels than is used for diagnosis can produce cell damage. These high power levels have been used for the treatment of cancer and by physiotherapists to treat muscle injuries. They should not be directed at the abdomen of a pregnant woman.

Despite its safety record, ultrasound should not be used unnecessarily; it is recommended for clinical benefit only. Most people would feel that to have an ultrasound examination merely to find out the sex of the fetus would be frivolous. If, however, a scan is being carried out for some other reason, then it takes little extra time to look at the sex if that is the couple's wish.

Neither you nor the fetus will notice any sensation from the ultrasound examination. In particular, the scan does not make you feel warm. As you do not feel anything, and you receive more power than the fetus since the ultrasound must pass through your tissues first, the fetus also cannot feel anything. Ultrasound cannot make the fetus move. Any movements observed during the examination are those that would have occurred naturally. There has also never been any evidence to support the suggestion that ultrasound can damage hearing.

THE EXAMINATION

The most vivid memory many women have of the scan is of an agonizingly full bladder. Fortunately this is now rarely necessary. An overfull bladder is in fact counterproductive, usually resulting in poor pictures. Check what your doctor wants you to drink. Often a little urine in your bladder is preferred but sometimes a totally empty one is best.

The logic of a full bladder was that it lifts the uterus out of your pelvis, sometimes making it easier to see through the abdomen. It also pushes the bowel, which contains air through which ultrasound waves will not pass, away from in front of the uterus. Modern equipment allows the operator to obtain good views without the woman having a full bladder by angling a small transducer through a part of the abdomen where intestines are not in the way.

When you lie on the examination couch for your ultrasound examination, some gel is squirted onto your abdomen — if you are lucky it will be warm. This gel allows the ultrasound to travel into your abdomen from the transducer. Without the gel there would be a thin layer of air between your skin and the transducer, which would reflect the ultrasound. As the transducer is only pressed gently on your abdomen, it will not hurt. It is moved around to produce images or sections through different parts of the fetus. At the completion of the scan the gel is wiped off.

If you need a scan in late pregnancy, you may have difficulty lying for a long period on your back. You may develop backache, feel uncomfortable, or become faint, dizzy, hot and sweaty. This is because the fetus and its amniotic fluid press on the blood vessels returning blood to your heart from your legs. If this happens tell the operator — it is best to turn onto your side and you will quickly feel better.

Vaginal Scan

This type of scan is also known as transvaginal (which means through the vagina) or endovaginal (which means in the vagina). A special transducer is gently passed into the vagina as you lie on your back with your legs bent up (see figure 3.5). The transducer, with its disposable cover, sits in the vagina, not in the uterus, so it can in no way harm a pregnancy or increase the risk of miscarriage. The transducer is cleaned after each use, and should then be soaked in a disinfectant solution, then wrapped in a clean, disposable cover for each patient so there is no risk of developing AIDS or other infections from the examination. A vaginal scan does not hurt. Most transducers are similar in size to one finger so they cause less discomfort than a gynaecological examination. Some people would prefer to pass the scanner themselves and there is no reason why you should not do this if you wish.

At first the idea of this scan is unpleasant and sounds uncomfortable. It is always your choice whether you have it performed. Of course you may refuse a vaginal scan, but don't forget that it would only be suggested if the doctor believed that it would allow more information to be obtained. A vaginal scan is more likely to be suggested if you are in early pregnancy. It has proved to be a major advance in the management of some complications, allowing them to be diagnosed earlier than was previously possible. It has been particularly useful in the early diagnosis of threatened miscarriage and tubal (or ectopic) pregnancy. You are likely to be given a much

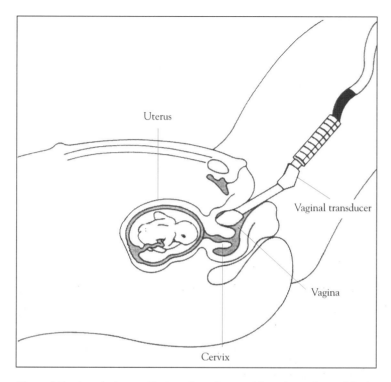

Uterus

Vaginal transducer

Vagina

Cervix

Figure 3.5 A vaginal scan: the transducer is passed into the vagina and 'looks through' the walls of the vagina and uterus at the fetus. Note that the transducer does not pass into the cervix or uterus, so it cannot disturb the pregnancy.

more accurate diagnosis in these situations than if the scan were performed through the abdomen.

Taking Along Your Partner or a Friend

During the scan you will be shown features of the fetus on the screen. You should also indicate whether you are planning to bring in your partner or other interested people. Most doctors are perfectly happy with this.

While many couples wish to include other children in the experience, this is not always successful. Children under six years of age cannot understand the scan with its two-dimensional 'slice of information' and may become restless. Finally, a warning — you will be surprised how many children think they will be taking the baby home with them after the scan.

Interpretation of the Picture

You will find the scan an exciting and rewarding experience but don't expect to understand every picture. Some views, such as a profile shot, are very straightforward, but others will be difficult or impossible for the inexperienced eye to interpret. You must keep in mind that you are looking at sections of the fetus and so will see the internal organs, not just the external appearance. A cross-section of the head is therefore not a view from above but rather a circle — the skull — with the inside of the brain visible within.

It takes years of practice to be able to fully interpret ultrasound pictures. You will mostly understand only the features pointed out to you. It is impossible for the operator to point out everything as well as concentrate on assessing fetal development. While doctors are aware that one of the joys of the ultrasound examination is that it enables you to relate to your unborn baby, it is also important as the first medical check.

The picture is presented as white on a black background. Solid tissue, such as bone, is seen as densely white, soft tissue as a lighter grey, and water or fluid as black. Hence the skull and long bones of the arms and legs are easy to see. The fetal bladder (which contains urine), the stomach (which contains fluid swallowed from the amniotic cavity), and blood in the heart look black. The amniotic fluid around the fetus also looks black (see the ultrasound images in chapter 4).

As you look at the screen, the top of the picture is your skin and the bottom is deep into your body. The left of the picture may be your left or right, head or feet end, depending on which way the transducer is orientated. The picture can be magnified, with centimetre marks down the side of the screen indicating the size of the picture in relation to actual size. In general what you see on the screen is beneath where the transducer touches you — if you see the head when the transducer is low on your abdomen then the head is lowermost in your body (figure 3.6).

If the fetus is facing upwards, the operator can show you a lifelike profile view (figure 3.7). If, however, it is facing away towards your spine, the face is hard to see and the picture looks much less human.

Strangely, you will find you can see much more human-looking pictures of the fetus earlier in pregnancy. At 10 or 12 weeks the tiny fetus usually will lie face up and the pictures can be quite beautiful. At 16 to 20 weeks wonderfully lifelike pictures can also usually be obtained. In the last three months of pregnancy, however, you are

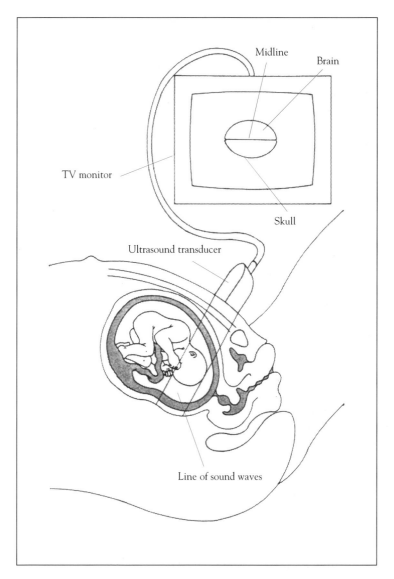

Figure 3.6 Producing an ultrasound picture: the ultrasound transducer sends out a line of sound waves through the tissues of the pregnant woman and the fetus. Small echoes from tissue layers reflect back to the transducer and are imaged on a TV monitor. As the transducer is over the fetal head a section (or slice) through the head is displayed — inside the skull, the brain and midline between the two halves of the brain are seen.

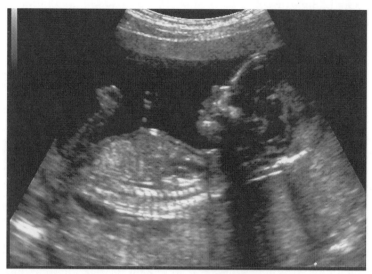

Figure 3.7 A profile view (head on right) with the fetus looking up. The nose, mouth and chin are visible. The cord is seen where it joins the abdomen, with the leg and knee on the left.

likely to be disappointed and find you cannot make out nearly as much detail (figure 3.8). At that time the fetus is too large for its entire image to fit onto the screen at one time. Each picture represents a thin slice of information from only a part of its anatomy and is thus hard to interpret.

Your own body build will alter the quality of the pictures. If you are plump, the layer of fat between the fetus and the transducer may prevent good pictures being obtained. Scars on your abdomen can also cause poor contact and result in poor pictures. Finally, the skill of the operator and the quality of the equipment will affect the clarity of the images.

A Picture to Take Home

'May I have a picture?' is undoubtedly the most frequent question asked. The answer is nearly always 'yes'. In this section we will look at the type of pictures available for you to take home and for the doctor's medical records (figure 3.9).

Polaroid film was initially used to record ultrasound images, but it has largely been replaced by thermal prints. Thermal prints are

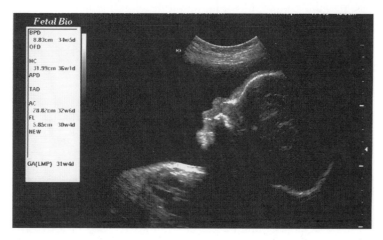

Figure 3.8 In the last three months ultrasound views of the fetus can be compromised both because of its size and the smaller volume of amniotic fluid. Unusually clear images of this 31-week fetus were obtained because it was lying face up and there was a relatively large amount of fluid present (the black area in front of its face).

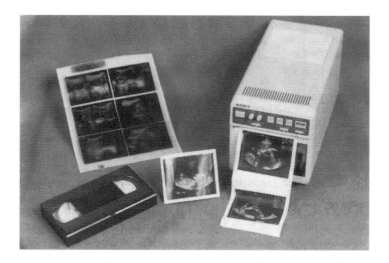

Figure 3.9 The types of pictures that can be produced using ultrasound — polaroid picture, X-ray film, video, thermal printer.

usually produced on cheap paper, similar to fax paper, but large, high-quality prints are also now available. Both polaroid and thermal prints will fade with time, especially if exposed to light, but they can be copied by a professional photographer if you want a long-lasting image.

The third option for a still record is a film similar to that used for X-rays. This is good for the doctors' records — high-quality, long-lasting, relatively cheap images — but not as acceptable to you for your unborn baby's first photograph.

Those looking for the ultimate record may desire a videotape of the fetus, preferably with commentary. There is some resistance amongst doctors to videotapes on several scores. It requires much more organization than a simple snapshot — a second video recorder (if the doctor uses one for his or her own records) or a constant change of tapes for successive patients. The provision of tapes may be difficult if the patient forgets to bring one. It should be pointed out that with so many distractions (taking a videotape for the family, recording pictures for the medical record, showing the pregnant woman and her family and friends on the screen), many doctors are worried that mistakes are more likely in the most important area a check of the fetus. Medico-legal considerations increasingly occupy the minds of the medical profession — there is some concern that the videotape may be used as a weapon against the doctor if things go wrong.

Questions

Is that ringing sound the ultrasound waves?

The noise that you hear is not the ultrasound waves. Some transducers make a ringing noise but this is machine noise. Ultrasound waves cannot be heard — they are above the range of human hearing.

Is ultrasound an X-ray?

No. No X-rays are used during an ultrasound examination. Ultrasound involves sound waves only. These are similar to those of speech so they do not have the potential problems of X-rays.

Do the sound waves make the fetus move?

Even though you might see only the fetus on the screen, the sound waves have in fact passed through you first. You receive far more of the ultrasound power than the fetus. Neither you nor the fetus feel anything, nor does the ultrasound stimulate movement. Those movements you see on the screen are the natural movements of the fetus in the uterus. Usually during the course of any scan after 9 weeks you will see at least some fetal movements.

Does ultrasound hurt the fetal ears?

No ill effects of ultrasound have been found at the power levels used for diagnosis. Doctors would not do scans if they thought the ultrasound waves could damage the ears, or other organs, of the developing fetus. Ultrasound used for diagnosis is believed to be safe.

Must I have a vaginal scan?

It is always your option to say no to any medical treatment that is offered to you. Usually a vaginal scan would only be offered if it is likely to provide better information. This is most likely to happen early in pregnancy.

Is that circle a picture of the head from above?

As shown in figure 4.3, the picture is not taken from above, but represents a thin slice of tissue. The circle therefore represents an image of the skull around the outside with the softer echoes of the brain within. It is as if you sliced through the fetal head and looked at the sliced end.

Why is my picture not as good as those of my friends?

The picture you are given depends on the stage of pregnancy and the way the fetus is facing. A profile view can often be obtained, which produces the most human-looking image, but this is not always possible. Also, the better the ultrasound machine, the better the picture is likely to be.

Can you still see through the fetus?

On seeing the internal organs of the fetus during an ultrasound examination, some people have the misconception that fetuses in early pregnancy are transparent. While they do have thin skin, you cannot see through them. Just as ultrasound travels through your tissues to get to the fetus, it also travels through the fetal skin to provide an image of its insides.

Where are the arms and legs on my picture?

A picture for you to keep is usually taken to include the fetal head and body. It is not possible to include all the arms and legs in the same slice.

Will I be able to listen to the heartbeat?

Ultrasound equipment includes technology that allows you to hear the fetal heartbeat. The equipment used to examine your pregnancy produces a picture on a television monitor so you can see the heartbeat, but unless there is some medical value in listening to it, this is not usually done.

What Ultrasound Can Show You

Although couples are able to obtain magnificent images of their unborn baby during an ultrasound examination, some are still unsure whether abnormalities are able to be detected with this method. This chapter explains those structures of the fetus that can be seen with ultrasound. It is possible to detect an abnormality in the development of any structure or organ than can be seen clearly, and the clearer the view, the more likelihood there is of even minor abnormalities being detected. This chapter emphasizes that if a structure can be seen clearly on a scan, and it looks normal, there is unlikely to be a major abnormality.

WHAT ABNORMALITIES ARE LOOKED FOR?

Irrespective of the reasons for your ultrasound examination, it is normal to examine the entire pregnancy — the fetus, amniotic fluid and placenta — as well as the uterus, and your pelvis for lumps. Areas particularly relevant to your situation are always examined in special detail, such as the fetal spine if you have previously had a baby with spina bifida.

It should be emphasized that not all abnormalities can be detected with ultrasound. Ultrasound shows *structure*, and an organ's structure may appear normal, but the organ may be disordered in function: for example, intellectual disabilities commonly occur in infants who have normally structured brains. The contrary also holds, in that the structure may appear grossly abnormal but produce only minor difficulties to the baby after birth. For example, a fetus with exomphalos (or a defect in its abdominal wall) may have a large structural abnormality but after birth a simple operation will result in a perfectly normal child. Some very mild defects may indicate a more severe abnormality elsewhere; for example, a fetus with overriding fingers may have a chromosomal abnormality.

Which abnormalities can be detected at an ultrasound examination depends greatly on the stage at which the pregnancy is scanned and any technical difficulties encountered at the time. Unfortunately, an abnormality that is readily diagnosed if the fetus is lying in one position may be difficult or impossible to diagnose if it is facing the opposite direction. A small heart abnormality or a cleft lip may be visible if the fetus faces up, but not if it faces down. In the best hands, however, ultrasound can detect an abnormality in up to 1 per cent of fetuses. Many more types of abnormality can be detected with ultrasound than with the more invasive tests such as amniocetesis and chorionic villus sampling (CVS).

WHEN IS THE BEST TIME?

Eighteen to 20 weeks is often chosen as the best time for an ultrasound examination because:

(i)   it is early enough to enable the due date to be calculated with sufficient accuracy in most pregnancies;

(ii) at this time the fetus is far enough advanced for most normal structures to be clearly visible;

(iii) if an abnormality is discovered it is early enough to have the pregnancy terminated if this is the couple's wish.

This is not the best time for an ultrasound examination for everybody. Women who have a complication either of this pregnancy or a previous one may well have an ultrasound examination much earlier. Those who have previously delivered a baby with hydrocephaly (water on the brain) or dwarfism may have an ultrasound examination a little later, as their measurements may remain within normal limits at 18 weeks.

WHY IS A SCAN SO IMPORTANT?

Obstetricians are increasingly offering an ultrasound examination to check the structure of the fetus. The advantages of doing so are as follows:

(i)   It provides enormous reassurance to parents. Most couples worry a great deal about the normality of the fetus. The reassurance of seeing normal structures, plus the added bonding that a normal ultrasound examination provides, is reason enough for the examination for many people.

(ii) If a significant abnormality is present, a couple may decide to have the pregnancy terminated. Couples who decide to continue the pregnancy have the advantage of being forewarned of the abnormality.

(iii) The knowledge that an abnormality is present allows medical staff to be forewarned. Some of the abnormalities detected on ultrasound may require urgent treatment at birth if the baby is to have the best chance of healthy survival. This often means that delivery should take place at a hospital where specialists and paediatric facilities are available.

(iv) It is sometimes important to know that an abnormality is present to allow a delivery to be brought on early, thus helping to minimize the continuing damage from that abnormality prior to birth. If ultrasound detects blocked kidneys, for example, and the condition deteriorates, the baby could be delivered early and the disease treated.

(v) There are occasional, albeit rare, abnormalities which may be treated prior to birth. Some of these are described in chapter 11.

MINOR ABNORMALITIES

The sensitivity of ultrasound equipment now also enables many minor variations from the norm to be detected. Unfortunately it is difficult to convince a couple whose fetus is shown to have an abnormality that it will only be minor. It can be very difficult for couples to keep such a finding in perspective. The widespread belief today that it is a couple's right to be fully informed of even the most minor abnormality can produce heightened anxiety over an insignificant defect. Some of the minor abnormalities relatively commonly identified on ultrasound, such as misshapen (club) feet and mild hydronephrosis (fluid on the kidneys), will be discussed in this section. For a more complete discussion on the structure of and abnormalities that can occur in a developing fetus, *Prenatal Diagnosis of Congenital Anomalies* by Romero, Pilu, Jeanty, Ghidini and Hobbins is recommended (see Further Reading).

DOWN SYNDROME

As most fetuses with Down syndrome have no major structural abnormalities, the condition cannot readily be detected on ultrasound at 18–20 weeks. After birth they exhibit some subtle facial differences, but these cannot be detected with a scan. The fetus may, however, have heart abnormalities or a blockage in the upper part of the intestines, which may sometimes be identified. When an abnorm-ality is detected with ultrasound, it is usually suggested that the chromosomes be tested to exclude the presence of Down syndrome and other chromosome abnormalities.

Efforts have been made to discover more subtle signs of Down syndrome. The first suggested sign was that the fetal head was more likely to be circular in shape, rather than the elongated shape of a normal skull. This has not proven to be a useful sign.

The second sign is known as nuchal oedema, and refers to a swelling in the tissues at the back of the neck (figure 4.1). Nuchal oedema has been associated with Down syndrome. At around 10 to 13 weeks, the removal of fluid from beneath the skin at the back of

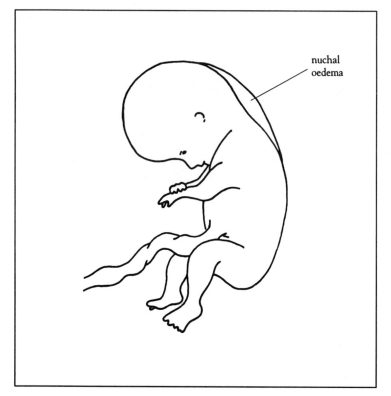

Figure 4.1 Diagram of a 10-week old fetus showing the swelling of the layer beneath the skin at the back of the neck, known as nuchal oedema.

the neck is inefficient, and all fetuses develop a thin fluid layer under the skin. With increasing thickness of this layer, there is an increasing risk of Down syndrome. The chance of Down syndrome rises with increasing thickness of the fluid layer and with the age of the pregnant woman. The cut-off point is around 3 mm, and detection rates for Down syndrome of up to 80 per cent have been reported. Whether or not the fetus has Down syndrome, this fluid layer usually absorbs during pregnancy, usually by 15 to 18 weeks, so it becomes a less reliable sign. Nuchal oedema is not a true abnormality and, except in severe cases, the baby looks normal at birth. If nuchal oedema is found to be present with ultrasound the pregnant woman is offered chromosomal testing for Down syndrome, such as amniocentesis or CVS. If the chromosomes of the fetus are normal it is uncommon for there to be any other abnormality, particularly if the nuchal thickness is only 3 or 4mm. Nuchal oedema is further discussed in chapter 8.

Many other signs of Down syndrome have been reported, although these are less accurate and would not normally justify any extra tests, unless more than one sign is present. They include:
(i)   slightly shortened long bones
(ii)   an in-curved fifth finger
(iii) a small bony centre in the middle section of the fifth finger
(iv)   increased fluid within the collecting system of the kidneys (pyelectasis)

No sign observable using ultrasound will indicate for certain that a fetus does have Down syndrome. These signs merely raise the index of suspicion — confirmation requires CVS, amniocentesis or fetal blood sampling to assess the chromosomes.

ULTRASOUND SECTIONS

Ultrasound is used to produce a series of sections through the fetus to visualize various structures and organs. The diagram in figure 4.2 shows where each of the ultrasound sections is taken. Although these structures can be seen from around 13 weeks, ultrasound examinations are commonly delayed until 18 weeks to enable better views.

Head and Spine

Figure 4.3 shows a section high up in the head with the skull encasing the brain. Note that it is a slice through the tissues of the skull and brain so that the structure of the brain itself is visible. It is not a

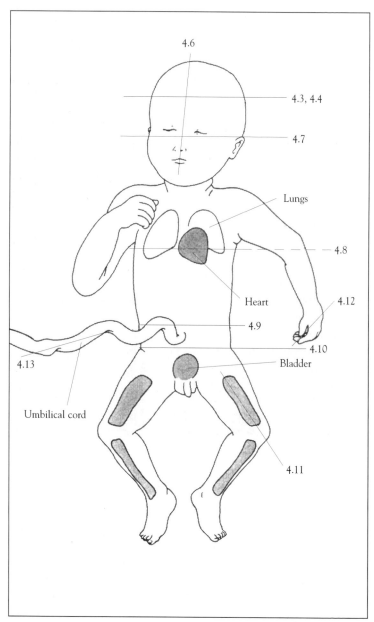

Figure 4.2 Each of the lines corresponds to the level to which each of the figures in this chapter was taken.

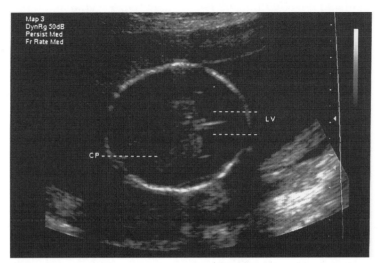

Figure 4.3 The head, showing the two fluid-filled chambers of the brain (LV = lateral ventricles). The fluid in the ventricles is produced by blood vessels in the choroid plexus (CP).

view from above the head. This section is carefully examined as it contains the midline between the two hemispheres of the brain, as well as the lateral ventricles, which are the main fluid-containing chambers. Three important abnormalities can be detected using this section.

Anencephaly is a condition in which the bony skull and most of the brain is absent. It is readily identified as the structures normally seen in the section through the head and brain are all missing. There is no treatment, and the baby dies before or immediately after birth. The incidence of anencephaly varies throughout the world between 0.5 and two per 1000 births. It is most common in Ireland and Wales and uncommon in Asian countries.

Hydrocephaly is an increase in the amount of cerebrospinal fluid in the chambers of the brain. Occurring in 0.5 to three births per 1000, it is diagnosed when the size of the ventricles is larger than expected. Hydrocephaly is often associated with other abnormalities and is present at birth in nearly all babies with spina bifida. After birth hydrocephaly is treated by placing a tube (a shunt) from the enlarged ventricles to the abdomen to drain the fluid. Prior to birth, hydrocephaly can be treated by a drainage procedure, but the results of this technique suggest that it does little to reduce the damage from the condition. The outlook for hydrocephaly depends on its cause and severity. Severe hydrocephaly detected prior to birth has a very poor outlook.

Choroid plexus cysts, shown in figure 4.4, are small pockets of fluid that become trapped within a collection of tiny blood vessels, called the choroid plexus, which is situated within the brain. These cysts are not present in the brain substance itself, and

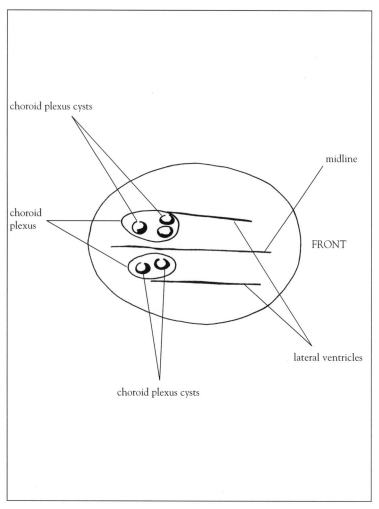

Figure 4.4 Choroid plexus cysts are pockets of fluid that lodge within a collection of blood vessels in the brain. They do not form in the brain substance itself.

therefore do not cause brain damage, cerebral palsy, or intellectual impairment. In addition, they do not grow during the pregnancy. Since the cysts themselves never cause any problem, they do not need to be checked again — they usually disappear by around 24 weeks. Choroid plexus cysts are seen in at least 1 in 100 fetuses scanned at 18 to 20 weeks.

The only reason to take notice of choroid plexus cysts is because they occur frequently in fetuses with an extra chromosome 18 — an abnormality known as Trisomy 18. Babies born with Trisomy 18 usually die shortly after birth. Most have other abnormalities, particularly in the heart and limbs, so when a choroid plexus cyst is detected a scan should be carried out by an experienced operator using state-of-the-art equipment who is skilled in examining these structures. If such a scan reveals no other abnormality, there is rarely any significance in the choroid plexus cyst. The chance of Trisomy 18 being present is linked to the age of the pregnant woman, but it is small compared to the normal risks of pregnancy. For example, the risk of Down syndrome carried by a pregnant woman at any specified age is greater than the chance of Trisomy 18 when the fetus is shown to have choroid plexus cysts but no other abnormality. Therefore, most pregnant women would not choose to have an amniocentesis for choroid plexus cysts alone. It is important not to think of the presence of choroid plexus cysts as an abnormality; it is merely a sign to look for other abnormalities.

A section of the whole length of the spine can be seen in figure 4.5. It normally shows each of the vertebra bodies and the overlying skin. In the presence of **spina bifida**, there is usually a lack of skin and an absence of the back wall of the vertebrae in the affected segment of the spine. This condition is covered in greater detail in the following chapter.

Face and Neck

In figure 4.6 the fetal nose, lips and chin are visible in profile. Figure 4.7 shows the eyes and the bridge of the nose. A lower section will show the line of the upper jaw, the overlying lip and, at the back, the lower part of the skull in the region of the back of the neck.

The face is examined to assess the size of the eye sockets and the features of the profile and mouth. **Facial clefts** are the most common abnormality in this area, estimated to occur in approximately one in 1000 births. Most of these involve the lip alone or the lip and the underlying palate. If the palate alone is affected it is usually further back in the mouth and unlikely to be diagnosed on ultra-

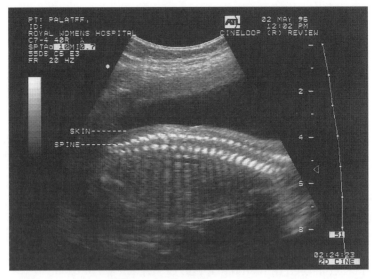

Figure. 4.5 The two parallel lines are the bones of the spine. The overlying skin is clearly visible above them.

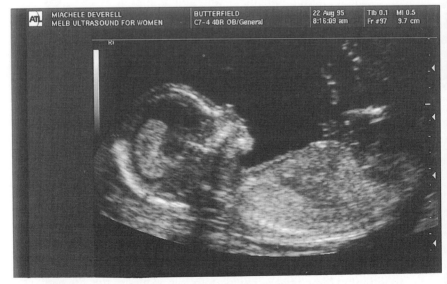

Figure 4.6 A profile view of the fetus showing the nose, lips and chin. Loops of cord are visible in front of the abdomen.

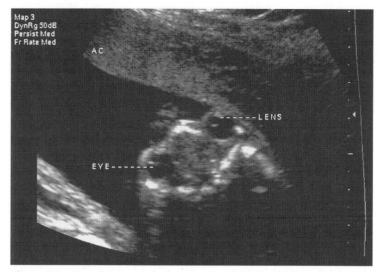

Figure 4.7 A section across the face showing the eyes (the lens of the eye is visible as a small white ring). The bridge of the nose can be seen between the two eyes.

sound. With satisfactory views of the face, many with a cleft lip and palate may be detected, but the smaller lesions may be difficult or impossible to see. If this is the only abnormality then a good cosmetic result can be expected with current surgical techniques.

Cystic swellings around the neck of the fetus, known as cystic hygromas, occur in approximately one in 200 pregnancies that miscarry, but are uncommon in liveborn babies. These are readily diagnosed on ultrasound. The outlook for the fetus depends on the degree of swelling of the neck and whether there is swelling else where in the body. This condition may indicate a chromosomal abnormality, most commonly Turner syndrome (see chapter 5).

Heart and Lungs

In the cross-section of the fetal chest shown in figure 4.8 the four chambers of the heart are visible. If other sections are also taken around the heart then the vessels entering and leaving the heart may also be examined.

There are a large number of structural abnormalities of the heart and they occur in at least one in 125 births. Many of these are not detectable prior to birth. This is a difficult area of diagnosis that requires equipment with excellent resolution and an experienced

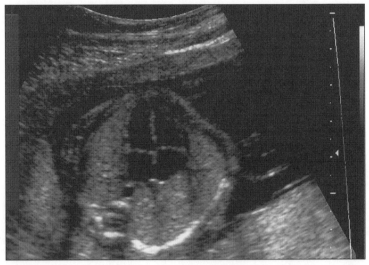

Figure 4.8 A cross-section of the chest showing the four chambers of the heart. The white areas around the heart are the lungs (the spine is at 7 o'clock).

operator. Under these conditions, however, it is now possible to detect at 18 weeks almost half of those fetuses with a heart abnormality. Advances in cardiac surgery have meant that babies who would have previously died of the heart abnormality may now be treated surgically after birth. If a heart abnormality is detected with ultrasound it is usually recommended that the chromosomes be tested.

Abnormalities of the lungs prior to birth are rare. The most common is cysts on one lung, which is diagnosed when a localized fluid collection is seen beside the heart. Even if moderately large, these can commonly be removed after birth, often with an excellent outlook. Occasionally they need to be drained prior to birth.

Abdomen and Abdominal Wall

The section shown in figure 4.9 is the most important one for checking the growth of the fetus. Deficiencies in the skin and muscle of the abdominal wall may lead to some of the contents developing outside the abdomen. There are two conditions: **exomphalos**, where there is a lining over the bulge, and **gastroschisis**, where there is no lining. Together these occur in approximately one in 5000 births. They are usually readily diagnosed on ultrasound and require no treatment

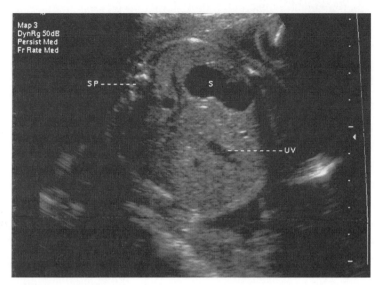

Figure 4.9   A section through the middle of the abdomen. The umbilical vein (UV) is visible on its way from the cord to the heart (Sp=spine, S=stomach).

prior to birth. Most can be closed after birth with a most successful outcome. Some of the fetuses with an exomphalos may also have other associated abnormalities, which may be detected with ultrasound or by chromosomal analysis.

Diaphragmatic hernia is a deficiency in the diaphragm, which causes some of the contents of the abdomen to ride up into the chest. The hernia is most commonly on the left side of the diaphragm with the stomach becoming positioned in the chest. This type is often diagnosed on ultrasound but some of the other types are more difficult. The hernia can be surgically treated at birth, but the major problem is that the presence of abdominal contents in the chest constricts the growth of the lungs. This is difficult to test prior to birth, but after birth it may be found that the lung development is inadequate for the baby's survival.

Kidney abnormalities

The kidneys represent one of the more difficult diagnostic areas. They may be seen early in pregnancy, but it is their function that is of prime importance. Function is assessed by the presence of urine in the bladder and the amount of amniotic fluid, most of which comes from the fetal urine. The absence of amniotic fluid prior to birth usually results in inadequate lung development to sustain life after birth.

Kidney abnormalities occur in approximately 0.8 per cent of babies. These include absence of one or both kidneys, cysts, and blockage of the outflow of urine. Some of these abnormalities result in death either before birth or immediately after. Those fetuses with a blockage of the outflow below the level of the kidneys may occasionally be suitable for treatment by inserting a tube above the level of the blockage to drain into the amniotic space (see chapter 11).

Hydronephroses is an enlargement of the collecting system of the fetal kidneys. It is usually due to a blockage somewhere in the outflow from the kidneys.

Pyelectasis is the word used to describe a small increase in the amount of fluid in the collecting system of the kidney (see figure 4.10). Urine from the kidney passes into a collecting chamber in the kidney known as the pelvis (not to be confused with the bony pelvis at the hips). In normal fetuses some urine can be seen in each plevis, the upper limit of normal being approximately 3mm. However, if the measurement is 4mm or more, there is not necessarily a problem —

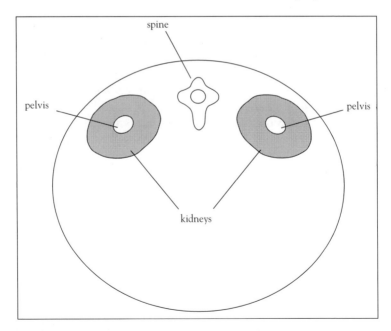

Figure 4.10 Pyelectasis is an increased volume of fluid within the collecting system (or pelvis) of each kidney.

it can simply be a normal variation in size. If the measurement is between 4 and 10 mm, the fetus rarely develops any problem before birth. Some develop vesico-ureteric reflux later in childhood, that is, every time they pass urine, some also flushes back up the tubes (the ureters) towards the kidneys. These children may need treatment with antibiotics and occasionally, if it is severe, surgery, but if the condition is recognised early, there is rarely any long-term damage.

The proportion of fetuses with pyelectasis that develop subsequent problems is unclear, so it is difficult to know whether to do tests on these babies after birth. Depending on the amount of fluid seen in the pelvis on the scan, another scan later in the pregnancy may be advised. Occasionally the pelvis continues to enlarge during the pregnancy, but it is uncommon for it to enlarge enough to cause kidney damage, so it rarely changes management of the pregnancy.

It has been suggested that fetuses with an increased amount of fluid in the pelvis at around 18 weeks are at higher risk for Down syndrome. This is an uncommon association, and the exact frequency is unknown, so unless there are other signs of Down syndrome, this alone would not usually be considered a reason to test with amniocentesis or CVS.

Fetuses with a small amount of fluid in the collecting system of the kidney rarely have a significant problem. It is often worthwhile checking progress with a scan in later pregnancy, and perhaps with investigations after birth, but the outlook is usually excellent.

Limbs

During an examination of the fetus each of the limbs is inspected. As calcium starts to form in the bones by the end of the third month of pregnancy, bones stand out as dense white lines. The soft tissues, such as muscles, are seen around the bone in figure 4.11. It is usually a simple matter to measure the length of any long bone, that of the thigh (femur) being the commonest.

Dwarfism is diagnosed if the length of the bones in the limbs is below the normal range. The diagnosis may be made as early as 14 to 16 weeks, but may not be possible until as late as 22 weeks. The limbs of fetuses affected by dwarfism increasingly fall below the normal range as pregnancy advances. While some babies with dwarfism, although short, lead a normal life, there are a large number who also have abnormalities in other regions of the body. In such cases, the baby may not survive after birth.

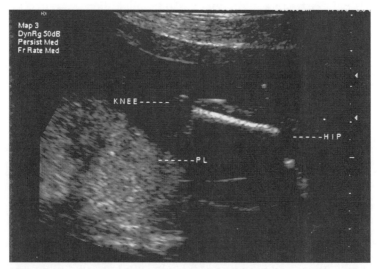

Figure 4.11 A section along the length of the thigh showing the femur (the bone) as a dense white line. The ends of the femur do not have bone laid down in them so they are not easily visible (PL=placenta).

Bone fractures may occur prior to birth in conditions such as **osteogenesis imperfecta** (brittle bones). In this condition the bones break very easily and may be markedly bent prior to birth.

Feet and Hands

The feet are readily seen on ultrasound and may be checked to ensure that each foot is at the appropriate angle to the lower part of the leg. Club feet, if severe, may be detected prior to birth as the foot is twisted around on the lower leg.

Figure 4.12 shows the hands and fingers. It is usually easy to count the fingers, but depending upon the position of the hand it may also be very difficult. Therefore, extra or missing fingers may at times be difficult to see. In addition, abnormalities in the shape of the hand or position of the fingers are occasionally detected.

Umbilical Cord

The umbilical cord is seen in figure 4.13 as a chain-like structure. If a section is taken across the cord the three vessels may be seen within it. Pregnant women often ask if it is possible to see whether the cord is around the neck of the fetus. This can be seen, but it is very common and rarely causes any complication. It is likely to be associated with difficulties at delivery only if it wrapped tightly around the neck several times.

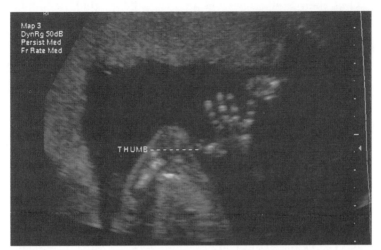

Figure 4.12   The bony centre in each of the segments of each finger is visible.

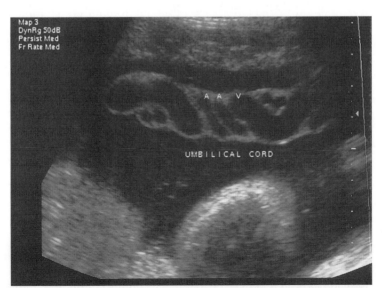

Figure 4.13   The umbilical cord showing the three blood vessels: two arteries (A) and one vein (V).

ERRORS AND PSEUDO-ERRORS

Ultrasound cannot detect all abnormalities in all fetuses. Anybody can make errors and this certainly happens with ultrasound. Simply because there is a complication of pregnancy does not mean that it should have been diagnosed by ultrasound. Before you accept that ultrasound 'missed' a complication, consider each of the following factors:

(i) Was the scan performed at an appropriate time to diagnose that complication? For example, in the first two and a half months of pregnancy few abnormalities can be detected. Even late in pregnancy one or two limbs or the spine may be virtually impossible to see properly.

(ii) Because an abnormality is severe, it is not necessarily readily detected. A port-wine stain on the face may be unsightly but would not be detectable on ultrasound. As mentioned above, Down syndrome in most fetuses may also be missed.

(iii) The position of the fetus at the time of the scan affects the ability to detect abnormalities. If it is lying face up, the spine may be difficult to see properly but the face and chest are likely to be clearly visible. If it is lying face down, the heart and face may be masked but beautiful views of the spine obtained. The fetus will often turn during the scan so that all of it may be seen well, but this does not always happen.

(iv) An abnormality might be seen but the cause of it misinterpreted. A cyst in the abdomen may be part of the bowel, in which case it is usually of no consequence to the baby, or it may be blocked kidneys, with the most dire consequences.

(v) Expectations as to what may be detected at your scan depend on the equipment used, the skill of the doctor, and the build of the woman having the scan. It is much harder to see clearly if the woman is obese or has surgical scars on the abdomen.

OVER-DIAGNOSIS

Over-diagnosis can be as important as under-diagnosis. The anxiety suffered by couples who are told that their fetus has a problem, no matter how minor, only to find out later that it is normal, cannot be overestimated. For example, one well-recognized abnormality diagnosed is fluid on the kidney — hydronephrosis. Many a pregnant woman has been told that the fetus has a hydronephrosis, when it is only a small, normal amount of fluid in the kidney's collecting system, which later disappears without treatment.

In the first three months of pregnancy it is also normal for the skin of the abdomen to be open with the intestines developing outside. If noted then, this should not be called an abnormality as the intestines later return into the abdomen. If the finding is present at four months, however, it is undoubtedly abnormal.

A low-lying placenta early in pregnancy can also cause a false alarm. Couples have been known to cancel overseas trips because the placenta looked low on ultrasound, only to find later that it was normal and did not prove to be a problem.

Questions

Can I trust my doctor to tell me everything?
Doctors today usually believe in telling their patients about any complication of pregnancy. If you are concerned that you are not being given the full story, then ask, but important facts are rarely kept from pregnant women. It is possible you will not receive the results of your scan on the day it is actually performed. Technicians are often restricted in the information they can give to patients and are usually not permitted to counsel them. There is never any problem in asking in advance whether you will receive complete information at the time of your scan or whether you will have to wait until you return to your obstetrician.

Why can't I see as much as I could early in pregnancy?
Strangely, you will find it harder to make out the features of the fetus later in pregnancy than you could in the early stages. The fetus becomes too large to fit readily on the ultrasound screen and is less likely to lie in a position that allows a life-like profile view to be obtained.

What abnormalities can ultrasound detect?
In a book such as this it is impossible to list all the abnormalities that may be detected in a fetus. The general principle is that every time you see a normal structure, some abnormalities are excluded. This chapter gives you an idea of some of the more common abnormalities which can be found.

Can the fingers and toes be counted?
Yes, but it may be difficult.

Causes of Fetal Abnormalities

If you wish to make a fully informed decision about prenatal testing then you need an overall understanding of the causes of abnormalities. There is a tendency to believe that the only important ones are Down syndrome and spina bifida. While these are very important, they are just two of an array of mostly rare conditions a newborn baby can have. In this chapter we will look at the wider picture of genetic abnormalities, what causes them, how common they are, and which can be detected before birth.

THE CHROMOSOMES AND GENES

Before looking at specific abnormalities, it is important to have some understanding about the chromosomes and genes. Cells of the fetus collected during procedures such as amniocentesis and CVS are most often tested for chromosome and single gene abnormalities.

Humans have about 50 000 pairs of genes or inherited characteristics contained within 23 pairs of chromosomes, one in each pair is received from each parent (see figure 5.1). The same chromosomes and genes are present in every cell of the body. One chromosome pair determines the sex of the individual; females have two X chromosomes and males an X and Y. The remaining 22 pairs are called autosomes and, along with genes on the X chromosome, they determine the many characteristics of each human being, such as hair and skin colour, appearance, height and intelligence. Individual chromosomes contain hundreds of genes, as shown on figure 5.2, each of which represents in chemical code the information to allow the body to make one specific protein with a unique function. Each gene is located at a specific position on its chromosome and can be found at the same place in all people.

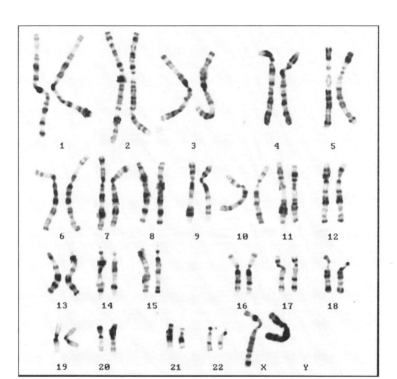

Figure 5.1 A chromosone analysis of a normal female fetus. There are 22 pairs of chromosomes, plus the two X chromosomes — a total of 46.

Testing Chromosomes before Birth

Both the cells that float in the amniotic fluid and those in the placenta are derived from the fetus. They have the same chromosome make-up as the fetus so they can be sampled for analysis. As only a few cells are shed into the amniotic fluid, a relatively large volume (around 15 ml) needs to be taken to find enough cells for reliable chromosome analysis. This method is known as amniocentesis. Chorionic villus sampling (CVS) involves the analysis of cells from the developing placenta (or chorion). Fetal blood is occasionally sampled from the umbilical cord or heart when there is doubt about the results of amniocentesis or if there is a need for quick results. Specimens can be taken from other parts of the fetal body, such as urine from the bladder, but this is rare.

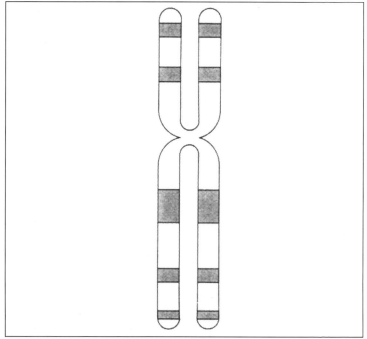

Figure 5.2 A diagram illustrating one of the 46 chromosomes in each cell. Each of the shaded areas is a gene which may be responsible for one characteristic (in reality each chromosome contains hundreds of genes). Often several genes are responsible for determining a single characteristic such as hair colour, colour of eyes, baldness etc.

CAN ALL ABNORMALITIES BE DETECTED BEFORE BIRTH?

It is estimated that about 4 per cent of liveborn babies have an abnormality, the cause of which is unknown in most. About 0.6 per cent have a chromosomal abnormality, 1 per cent have one of the 5000 or so rare single gene disorders and at least 2 per cent are born with a structural malformation. The latter are disorders such as spina bifida, heart malformations and cleft lip and palate, which are influenced by genes as well as unknown other factors. It is only the chromosome abnormalities, some of the single gene disorders and a few congenital malformations that can be detected by amniocentesis or CVS. As these make up only a small percentage of the possible problems, it is clear that the tests do not guarantee a normal baby. This is an important point because many women regard a normal result on the tests as a stamp of normality on the fetus. There are other more common problems associated with pregnancy, such as prematurity, which occurs in about one in 20 births. In addition, about 10 per cent of fetuses grow poorly in the last half of pregnancy, with increased risk of complications occurring.

Intellectual disability is probably the most feared abnormality. It is estimated that about one in 200 (0.5 per cent) newborn infants are severely or profoundly intellectually disabled. Many die early so that by the age of five, 0.3 to 0.4 per cent of children are intellectually impaired. Estimates vary on the contribution of causes. At the most, 40 per cent of intellectual disability is due to a chromosome abnormality and might be detected before birth. Down syndrome is by far the most common cause, followed by the fragile X syndrome, an inherited condition in which the X chromosome has a characteristic abnormality when seen through a microscope. Most of the remaining 60 per cent of intellectually disabled infants cannot be detected prior to birth. Some are the result of single gene disorders, others are the result of external factors such as infection or lack of oxygen before birth. At least a third of cases have no known cause.

With current rapid advances in medical genetics, the range of disorders amenable to prenatal diagnosis is likely to widen rapidly. It has only been possible in the last few years, for example, to diagnose haemophilia and cystic fibrosis prenatally. Currently, about 300 single gene defects can be detected, but not every pregnant woman can be screened for all the disorders for which tests exist — there are simply too many tests. Unless a fetus is at special risk of a particular disorder, invasive testing will only indicate whether the fetal chromosomes are normal and confirm the sex. Amniocentesis will also show whether there is a risk of spina bifida. If the fetus has any other abnormality, such as a new mutation, it would not be detected unless visible on ultrasound. In the best hands, ultrasound is likely to detect an abnormality in up to 1 per cent of fetuses, particularly many of the more serious structural conditions.

On the brighter side, of the 4 per cent of babies born with an abnormality, about half are not serious and include such conditions as a port wine stain or an extra toe.

SINGLE GENE DEFECTS

There are about 5000 recognized single gene defects, most very rare conditions, inherited from generation to generation. In the past, it has been difficult to diagnose such conditions prior to birth, even if a couple had a previously affected child, because the fault may lie in one specific gene. The first to be diagnosed before birth were those conditions, such as metabolic disorders, which produce an abnormal substance that can be detected in the amniotic fluid or fetal blood.

The most recent major development in diagnosis is by direct analysis of DNA, the building blocks of chromosomes. Scientists throughout the world are now attempting to determine the actual site on the chromosome where each of the genes occur. As knowledge of the location of genes increases, some diseases which occur because of abnormalities in either one or small numbers of genes can be diagnosed by studying the chromosome itself. Some are detected by probes for the actual gene, but more often it is nearby marker genes that are tested.

Prenatal analysis is not normally carried out unless there is a history of a disorder in the family, or the couple already has an affected child. In such cases, a geneticist will be able to tell you the chance of a defective gene being passed on to your baby and whether it is likely to cause any major problems. This is because gene defects follow clearly defined patterns of inheritance, first outlined in the nineteenth century by an Austrian monk, Gregor Mendel.

Put simply, each parent contributes a gene for a particular characteristic to each of their children. Normal genes and gene defects may be dominant or recessive. For dominant conditions, such as Huntington's disease, carriers of one copy of the gene defect will develop the disease. An affected parent will then have a one in two chance of passing it on to each of his or her children. Most conditions, however, are recessive and quite harmless to those who carry only one copy of the gene. For the disease to manifest, both parents must be carriers of the gene defect. The risk to each of their children is then one in four. Prenatal testing for couples with a family history or a child afflicted with such disorders can be of profound assistance and give them the courage to have a family.

While many single gene disorders produce seriously debilitating illnesses, they are also very rare, and their frequency varies between geographic regions. Some of the more common genetic diseases that can be diagnosed before birth are described below.

Cystic fibrosis is the most common single gene disorder among those of Northern European descent, affecting about one in 2000 liveborn babies. Cystic fibrosis is a condition that results in recurrent respiratory infections and is usually fatal in early adulthood. The recessive gene is carried by one in 20 people, upon whom it has no obvious impact. This condition could not be detected before birth until it was discovered that abnormal enzymes were present in the amniotic fluid. This enzyme test had some problems, however, because of borderline results. Gene probes have now been developed which can give most couples a definitive result at CVS. Population screening may one day become available by testing everyone's blood, so those couples at risk can be identified.

The red blood cell disorders known as **thalassaemias** cause major health problems in Italy, Greece, some of the Mediterranean islands, and parts of South-East Asia. Gene probes can be used to test for the disorder in most at-risk families. For the rest, fetal blood sampling can be done at 18 weeks to determine whether the fetus has inherited the gene defect from both parents. One copy of the gene has little impact, while two copies result in severe anaemia and shortened lifespan.

Testing is also now available for **Huntington's disease**, a dominant condition causing severe body movements plus mental deterioration after the age of 40. Those with relatives afflicted by the disease can be tested to find out if they will also develop it. The condition can also be diagnosed prenatally.

Haemophilia and Duchenne muscular dystrophy are **sex-linked conditions**, recessive gene disorders on the X chromosome, which are only likely to affect sons of women who are carriers. Each son will have a one in two chance of being born with the disease. Haemophilia is a bleeding disorder caused by the blood lacking a clotting factor. Usually couples with a high risk of a baby with haemophilia will be tested by CVS, but some require fetal blood sampling at 18 weeks. Muscular dystrophy results in increasing muscular weakness, commencing in early childhood and usually resulting in death in early adulthood. This may also be diagnosed using CVS.

CHROMOSOME ABNORMALITIES

A chromosome abnormality may be so minor that it produces no ill effects in the offspring or so major that it results in miscarriage very early in the pregnancy. About half of all miscarriages are associated with chromosome abnormalities. There can also be a large range of major and minor developmental defects between these two extremes. Those experienced at interpreting chromosomal abnormalities can usually tell what, if any, defect is usually associated with a particular chromosome abnormality.

The frequency of chromosome abnormalities at birth is about six in 1000. Of these, around a third result from rearrangements of chromosome material and the rest from variations in the number of chromosomes. Table 5.1 shows the more common chromosome abnormalities. Major abnormalities often result if there are more than the normal 46 chromosomes. Down syndrome, or Trisomy 21, in which there is an extra chromosome 21, is the most common chromosome abnormality to cause a major disability in children (see figure 5.3). Another relatively common trisomy, or condition with an extra chromosome, is Trisomy 18. It is associated with a number of major abnormalities and usually results in the child dying shortly after birth. Triploidy, where there are three of every chromosome, result-ing in a total of 69 chromosomes, usually results in a spontaneous miscarriage early in pregnancy.

Variations in the number of sex chromosomes make up about a third of the chromosome abnormalities found at birth. This is a range of conditions in which the baby has either fewer sex chromosomes than normal or extra copies of the X or Y chromosome. While it is possible to detect these prenatally, sex chromosome variations pre-sent couples with some of the most difficult decisions because their effects are less severe.

Another quite common chromosomal variation found at testing is mosaicism. This is a term used when an individual has some cells in his or her body with one type of chromosomal make-up and other cells with another type. This individual then has some of the features derived from each chromosomal type, the final characteristics depending on the relative proportions of each. A child with mosaic Down syndrome has a mixture of normal cells and those with an extra chromosome 21. Such babies will have some of the features of Down syndrome, but will be less severely affected. Chromosomal mosaicism is occasionally found in the placenta at CVS, in which case it is usually associated with a normal fetus with normal chromosomes.

Chromosomal Rearrangements

These result from breakages in the chromosomes. Sometimes two chromosomes will have simply swapped pieces and the total amount of chromosome material will be normal. This is called a balanced translocation and usually has no effect on the child. At other times, chromosome material will be lost or gained as a result of a chromo-some breakage. This situation is called an unbalanced chromosome translocation and is usually associated with intellectual impairment.

TABLE 5.1 INCIDENCE OF SOME OF THE MORE IMPORTANT
ABNORMALITIES IN LIVEBORN BABIES

Condition	Approx. incidence in 1000 births	Method of diagnosis	Proportion diagnosed
Chromosomal			
Down syndrome	1.5	Amnio/CVS	All
		U/sound	Some
Turner syndrome	0.2	Amnio/CVS	All
		U/sound	Some
XXX, XXY, XYY	1.0 each	Amnio/CVS	All
Single gene defects			
Cystic fibrosis	0.5	CVS	All in some families
Sex-linked conditions (e.g. haemophilia,* Duchenne muscular dystrophy (DMD))	0.5	Amnio CVS	Most All in some families
Neural tube defects			
Anencephaly	Varies	Amnio	All
		U/sound	All
Open spina bifida	Varies	Amnio	98%
		U/sound	Approx. 95%
Others			
Hydrocephaly	0.5–3	U/sound	Most, *after 20 weeks*
Cleft lip with or without palate	1.4	U/sound	Many, especially if severe
Heart abnormality	8	U/sound	Approx. $^{1}/_{3}$ including most of severe ones

Condition	Approx. incidence in 1000 births	Method of diagnosis	Proportion diagnosed
Abdominal wall deficiency	0.2	U/sound	Nearly all
Kidney abnormalities	8	U/sound	Most, especially if severe
Dwarfism	0.2	U/sound	Most, *after 20 weeks*
Club foot	1.2	U/sound	Many, especially if severe

Note: 1) Approximately 4 per cent of live newborns have an abnormality.
2) Except where stated the ultrasound is assumed to have been carried out at 18–20 weeks.
* Some families may need fetal blood sample for diagnosis.

When an unbalanced translocation is found on amniocentesis or CVS, the baby is highly likely to be abnormal and most couples decide to terminate the pregnancy. If a balanced translocation is detected, the chromosomes of the pregnant woman and her partner will be checked. Very often, one or other has the same balanced translocation and the baby can be expected to be healthy. If neither the woman nor her partner has the translocation there is a small chance that the child will be abnormal.

Down Syndrome

Down syndrome, previously called mongolism, is also known as Trisomy 21 because it is due to the presence of an extra chromosome number 21 in each cell. It is emphasized in antenatal diagnosis as it is the most frequent chromosomal abnormality resulting in a major disability in a surviving infant. Many of the other abnormalities produce either minor defects or such major ones that they result in death before or soon after birth. Children with Down syndrome are intellectually impaired and usually only reach an IQ of between 25 and 50, although with early education slightly higher scores may be

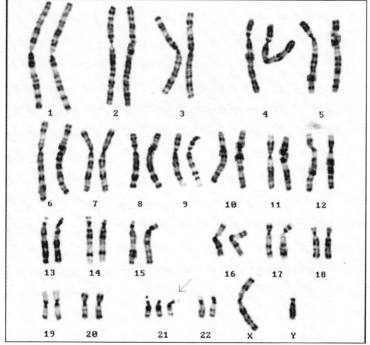

Figure 5.3 A chromosome analysis of a male fetus with Down syndrome. There is an additional chromosome 21, making a total of 47.

achieved. They are also likely to have any of a number of other abnormalities, for example, 40 per cent of those affected have a heart abnormality.

Down syndrome is present in one in 660 newborn babies. The majority of these occur 'out of the blue' to couples with no family history of chromosome abnormalities. The chance of having a baby with Down syndrome increases with the age of the pregnant woman, but the age of her partner has minimal influence (see figure 5.4). All of the eggs a woman produces during her lifetime are present in a primitive stage in the ovaries at the time of her birth. It is believed that with the passage of years, and the ageing of these eggs, there is an increased likelihood of chromosome abnormalities. It is important to realize that while the risk of having a Down syndrome baby increases with the pregnant woman's age, not all of the extra chromosomes 21 come from her. About one in 10 come from her partner.

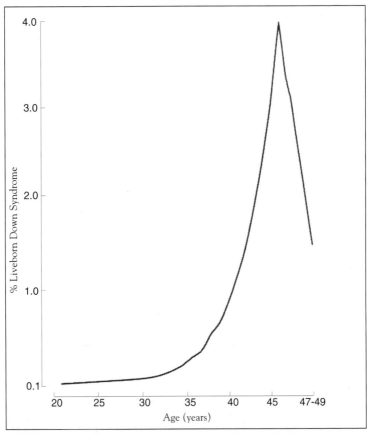

Figure 5.4 A graph showing the steep rise in incidence/likelihood of a Down syndrome baby with increasing age of the pregnant woman.

Table 5.2 shows a pregnant woman's chance of having a baby with Down syndrome at any given age. The left column shows the chance of a woman delivering a live baby with Down syndrome. The next column shows the chance the same woman has of having a Down syndrome fetus detected if she has an amniocentesis at 16 weeks. The third column shows the chance of a baby with any chromosomal abnormality being detected at the time of amniocentesis. The last two columns show the chance of these conditions being present at the time of CVS – 10 to 12 weeks. The figures are much higher in early pregnancy because Down syndrome fetuses have a very high miscarriage rate – of those present at 16 weeks, one in three will die before delivery.

TABLE 5.2 RISK OF CHROMOSOMAL ABNORMALITY

	LIVEBORN	AMNIOCENTESIS		CVS	
Age of pregnant woman	Down syndrome[1]	Down syndrome[2]	All unbalanced chromosome abnormalities	Down syndrome[3]	All unbalanced chromosome abnormalities
	One in:	One in:	One in:	One in:	One in:
21	1520				
23	1450				
25	1350				
27	1200				
29	1010	These figures are not available			
30	890				
31	775				
32	660				
33	545	420	200		
34	445	320	160		
35	355	280	120	240	115
36	300	250	100	205	85
37	220	180	80	155	65
38	165	135	65	115	50
39	125	100	52	85	39
40	90	75	42	65	30
41	70	60	33	45	22
42	50	45	26	35	17
43	40	35	20	25	13
44			17		10
45			14		8
46			11		6
47			8		4
48			6		3
49			5		

Sources: 1   Age 21–35: Hecht & Hook, *Prenat Diagn* 1994, 14, 729
   36+ Halliday, J. et al, *Prenat Diagn* 1995, 115, 455

   2   Age 21–35: Hook 1992, in *Prenatal Diagnosis and Screening*, Brock, Rodeck, Ferguson-Smith, et al., 351
   36+ Halliday, J. et al, *Prenatal Diagnosis*, 1995, 115, 455

   3   Hook, 1992, in *Prenatal Diagnosis and Screening*, Brock, Rodeck, Ferguson-Smith et al., 351

It is debatable which figures should be presented to couples. Which is the more important figure? Is it the chance of finding a Down syndrome fetus at amniocentesis or CVS when the couple will have to decide whether to accept an abortion? Alternatively, is it more important to tell a couple the chances of them delivering a live-born baby with Down syndrome for whom they will then be responsible? There is no uniformity on this issue, so all the figures are presented in table 5.2 for couples to use as they feel appropriate.

In the table the second column under both ammiocentesis and CVS shows the chance of a couple having a chromosome abnormality of significance detected at the time they have the test. These include both the serious ones, such as Trisomy 18, and the less serious ones, such as abnormalities of the sex chromosomes.

You will also notice that while information on liveborn babies is available down to 21 years of age, that on amniocentesis and CVS is not available below ages 33 and 35 respectively. This is because these tests have been offered on a regular basis only to 'older' women.

At first glance, one would imagine that most Down syndrome babies are born to older women, but this is not the case. It is estimated that 35 per cent (or approximately one in three) of Down syndrome babies are born to mothers of age 35 or above. If a testing program is used for women of 35 years and above, then two-thirds of the babies with Down syndrome would not be detected. This is because most women have their babies when they are young, so even though individually they are at low risk, collectively they produce more Down syndrome babies.

If a couple has previously had a baby with Down syndrome the chance of them having a second Down syndrome baby might increase. Under 30, the risk of a chromosome abnormality in each subsequent pregnancy is one in 100. Over 30, the risk is that associated with the age of the pregnant woman; that is, it is not increased.

There is a rare type of Down syndrome, called translocation Down syndrome, where the abnormality can run in families. As this is an uncommon problem (only 3 per cent of cases), we will not pursue it here. Its significance, however, is that the parents of a baby with this type of Down syndrome are tested to see if they have a rearrangement of chromosomes that puts them at extra risk. If they do, other family members may be at greater risk too.

Sex Chromosome Variations

Sex chromosome variations make up about a third of the chromosome abnormalities, and present couples with some of the most difficult decisions. This is because of the sometimes subtle abnormalities shown and the uncertain level of disability. Until the mid 1960s, knowledge about people with sex chromosome anomalies was based entirely on those who showed clinical symptoms, particularly intellectual impairment and disorders of behaviour. This provided a false view of sex chromosome abnormalities because only the most affected people were used to define the problems. Since then, large-scale screening of newborn infants has shown that 1 in 400 newborns has a sex chromosome variation, and we now know that most will live relatively normal lives.

Newborn chromosome surveys began in the mid 1960s and continued over the next decade with the aim of finding out what kind of effect sex chromosome variations have on development. Some 307 children were identified and followed up in seven studies of consecutive livebirths in the United States, Canada, Denmark and Scotland. Girls with an extra X chromosome and boys with either an extra Y or X were found to be the most common, with an incidence each of about one in every 1000 births.

Girls with an extra X chromosome (47XXX) are taller on average and may have delayed puberty. Two-thirds have normal intelligence, while a third have borderline IQ or intellectual impairment. Boys with an extra X chromosome (47XXY), a condition known as Kleinfelter syndrome, are also tall. They have a mild reduction in intelligence but have frequent specific learning problems. They are infertile and have delayed or incomplete puberty, which may be treated with hormones.

Boys with an extra Y chromosome (XYY syndrome) tend to be taller, are fertile, have normal intelligence and usually display normal behaviour. When the condition was first discovered, a higher incidence was found among prison inmates, leading to the conclusion that an extra Y chromosome predisposed carriers to aggressive and psychotic behaviour. Since then, follow-up studies have shown quite normal development in most, and the risk of behaviour problems seems to be lower than was first supposed.

A less common condition is Turner syndrome, the name given to the physical features of a girl with a missing X chromosome. The resultant sex chromosome pattern is called 45X. Turner syndrome occurs in about one in 5000 newborns. It is much commoner in early pregnancy, but most miscarry. Some Turner syndrome fetuses can be identified with ultrasound prior to birth. The features may include swelling of the tissues around the neck, fluid collection in other tissues, reduced amniotic fluid and poor growth. Such fetuses are very unlikely to survive until birth. When the fetus is less severely affected, for example minor swelling around the neck, this may subside during pregnancy and the fetus survive. If these features are detected with ultrasound, it is usual to check the fetal chromosomes. Only some will have Turner syndrome, others either having normal chromosomes or some other abnormality.

Newborn babies with Turner syndrome usually have less severe abnormalities. They may have webbing of the neck and an increased likelihood of heart and kidney abnormalities. While their intelligence is usually in the normal range, there may be some specific learning disabilities. Such children are of small stature and do not have functioning ovaries, so they cannot have children, except by using a donated ovum and in vitro fertilization technology.

Because genetic testing only tells you about the chromosomes, and not about the severity of any future disabilities, it can be quite confusing for parents considering what action to take. Although there have been large studies of children with sex chromosome variations, the range of possible outcomes is wide. The experiences of one couple, who found out at amniocentesis that their baby boy had Kleinfelter syndrome, illustrate the dilemma.

The outlook with Kleinfelter syndrome was not certain. Ben might simply be a tall, overweight, infertile person experiencing learning difficulties during middle childhood. Or he could be more severely intellectually disabled. He might develop secondary sexual character-istics only with the use of continued doses of hormones after puberty. But he might not. The literature suggested that he might have a predisposition to cancers of the testes or breasts. But it might not materialize. There was evidence of predisposition to psychotic illness. But he might be lucky. The information shifted and changed depending on what we read, the research methodology and who we spoke to.

If you are found to be carrying a fetus with a sex chromosome variation, you should see a specialist geneticist. He or she will have the latest information on the condition. About half the couples presented with this finding decide to terminate the pregnancy. Your decision will be based on your own family circumstances and expectations.

NEURAL TUBE DEFECTS (NTD)

Neural tube defects are malformations of the nervous system that have a strong genetic component, but the precise mode of inheritance is unknown. Inheritance of NTD is described as multifactorial — that is, it depends on a number of genes as well as external influences. All women planning to become pregnant should be aware that their chance of having a baby with a neural tube defect (that is, spina bifida or anencephaly) is reduced if they take folic acid supplements. This may also reduce the chance of the baby having some other abnormalities. All women planning pregnancy should take folic acid supplements for one month before conception and for six weeks following conception. Those at low risk of spina bifida should take 0.5mg of folic acid per day. Those at high risk should take 5mg of folic acid per day. It is available over the counter at your chemist or health food store. Couples at high risk include those who have had a previous baby affected by a neural tube defect and epileptics on treatment. The likelihood of a neural tube defect is reduced by about two-thirds if folic acid is taken as recommended above.

The incidence of neural tube defects varies throughout the world, the highest being in Northern Ireland, where one in 120 babies are affected. In Australia and the United States, it affects about one in 500, while in Japan the incidence is less than one in 1000. If a couple has had a previous baby affected with a NTD, or are affected themselves, the risk of it recurring in each subsequent pregnancy rises to about one in 30. If they do have a recurrence, the chances of it being either a spina bifida or anencephalic will be equal. **The incidence of NTD is not related to the age of the pregnant woman.**

There are two main types of neural tube defect: **anencephaly**, in which the skull and brain do not form properly; and **spina bifida**, in which part of the spinal column is open. Babies with anencephaly are stillborn or die shortly after birth because most of the brain is missing, while the problems caused by spina bifida depend on the size of the opening, its location and the amount of damage to the spinal cord and brain. If the defect is small, low in the spine, and covered by skin, there may be no problems or only mild difficulties with leg weakness and poor sensation. More often, the defect is large and not covered by skin. The spinal cord and its membranes may protrude through the opening and lie in a sac on the back. This often ruptures during pregnancy or at the time of delivery. The nerves to the lower part of the body, the legs, bladder and the bowel pass through the defect. If they are damaged, there is a variable degree of paralysis of the legs and loss of control of the bladder and bowel.

Babies with spina bifida also develop fluid on the brain (hydrocephaly) because they have an associated blockage to the flow of fluid from the brain. Varying degrees of intellectual impairment may occur, preventable in some cases by draining excess fluid through a shunt. Children with severe spina bifida may have a short lifespan. Some may be suitable for surgery to close the defect in the back. This protects against infection, but will not restore lost function.

Tests for Spina Bifida

Assessing the level of a substance known as alpha-fetoprotein (AFP) in the amniotic fluid was the first test developed for spina bifida. This is raised in about 98 per cent of affected fetuses. AFP is produced by babies prior to birth and is present in their bloodstream and spinal fluid. The level peaks at 13 weeks then decreases slowly until 40 weeks. If there is a defect in the skin, there will be a marked increase in the level of AFP that crosses to the amniotic fluid and pregnant woman's blood. The AFP level is usually tested in women having an amniocentesis in the first half of pregnancy. In some places all pregnant women are offered a test for AFP in their own bloodstream. This is discussed in chapter 8.

Another test which can also be carried out on amniotic fluid is for acetyl cholinesterase. When levels of this enzyme are also raised, it provides extra confirmation of an abnormality. CVS cannot be used to diagnose neural tube defects.

Ultrasound Diagnosis of NTD

Until recently all couples with a past history of spina bifida or anencephaly, and those with an unexplained elevation of maternal serum AFP, were offered amniocentesis. With increasing sophistication of ultrasound equipment this is now not always performed. After 16 weeks, ultrasound should diagnose about 95 per cent of spina bifida cases and all cases of anencephaly. A couple who have had a previous baby with spina bifida have a 1.5 per cent chance of anencephaly — all of which will be detected by ultrasound — and a 1.5 per cent chance of spina bifida. If the spine and head appear normal on ultrasound, using the above figures the risk of spina bifida falls to one in 1300. If the ultrasound is performed by an experienced operator who is able to obtain good views of the fetal head and spine, there is a good case for not proceeding with amniocentesis.

Additional reassurance can come from a normal maternal serum AFP result.

Apart from those with a previously affected baby, there are some other pregnant women who have a slightly higher than normal risk. These include couples who have a near relative with spina bifida and those on some medication, such as epileptics who are controlled on certain drugs. Many such couples have a risk of approximately one per cent of spina bifida being present in any pregnancy. Using the same logic as above, a normal ultrasound will miss a spina bifida in the fetus in only one in 5000 births. Ultrasound alone is therefore usually used for such couples, together with a maternal serum AFP test.

GENETIC COUNSELLING

Counselling about genetic diseases is available at several levels. It is generally your obstetrician who will discuss any appropriate prenatal tests with you. He or she will be able to tell you what increased risks you run because of your age or other factors, and indicate what tests are available, their risks and where expertise is available to have such tests. Some diagnostic centres offer formal genetic counselling sessions to all women considering testing. It is important that some form of information, written or verbal, provided by your obstetrician or counsellor, is available to you before you make any decisions.

Counselling sessions typically last about 30 minutes to an hour. More than two-thirds of couples seen for counselling are recommended because of the age of the pregnant woman These sessions will cover the chromosomes, the differences between amniocentesis and CVS, the risks of miscarriage from the procedures, and the risks of having a Down syndrome baby. The counsellor will explain the condition so that the woman has a full understanding of what her options are. Common misconceptions, such as the idea that you are at lower risk because you are healthy, or that bleeding in early pregnancy is a contra-indication to testing, will also be cleared up.

Another routine part of genetic counselling is the recording of a short family history. This is to make sure there are no other relevant inherited problems within the family of the pregnant woman or of her partner. For those having counselling for reasons such as the presence of a rarer genetic disorder, family histories are very important. The counsellor will need information about any illnesses affecting your parents and their brothers and sisters, as well as your own brothers and sisters and their children. If any previous pregnancies led to miscarriage or loss of the baby at birth or early in life, information about the cause, or the name of a doctor who may be able to provide details, will be needed. The counsellor will help determine what extra risks you, as a couple, have of producing a child with a specific genetic disease, and what this disease would mean for the affected child.

Such discussions will also be able to alleviate fears a woman might have about the impact of drugs taken before she realized she was pregnant. There is no evidence to indicate an increased birth defect risk with most commonly used medications.

After counselling, some women — particularly those who have suffered from infertility problems — are not prepared to place their pregnancy at any risk and decide not to go ahead with testing. Other couples are adamant about not bringing an abnormal baby into the world. Many women make the decision beforehand that they will terminate a pregnancy if the fetus has Down syndrome. It is important prior to undergoing testing to have a full understanding of what pregnancy termination would involve. With amniocentesis, for example, a termination is done at 18–20 weeks, usually by inducing labour, although in some centres it may be carried out surgically through the cervix by dilation and evacuation.

SUMMARY OF REASONS FOR TESTING

You are likely to be offered an amniocentesis or CVS if you fall within any of the following categories:

(i) Age of the pregnant woman is the major reason for testing, accounting for at least two-thirds of referrals. The precise minimum age at which women are offered tests varies, but is most commonly 35 years, sometimes taken at the date of the procedure and others times from the expected time of delivery. The age that is chosen depends on available local resources and the opinion of local experts. The flexibility of this 'minimum age' requirement also varies, the commonly held view now being that any couple should have access to counselling and prenatal testing, rather than having some arbitrary restriction.

(ii) A couple with a past history of a baby with a chromosome abnormality.

(iii)   A chromosome abnormality in either the pregnant woman or her partner.

(iv)   A woman who has had three or more miscarriages.

(v)   Subtle ultrasound findings which may mean there is an increased chance of a chromosome abnormality (see Chapter 4).

(vi)   Other ultrasound indications — these include significant structural abnormalities of the fetus, major reductions in its growth, and abnormalities of amniotic fluid volume.

(vii)   Abnormal results from biochemical tests on the pregnant woman — this includes an abnormal level of AFP and other such tests, as discussed in chapter 8.

(viii)   Some couples at high risk of having a baby with a neural tube defect, especially those who have previously had a baby with anencephaly or spina bifida, and those with a raised maternal serum AFP.

(ix)   Those couples with a single gene disorder, such as muscular dystrophy, haemophilia or thalassaemia in either family.

Questions

I have a close relative (e.g. sister, brother, cousin) with Down syndrome. What are my chances of having such a baby?

Your chances of having a baby with Down syndrome are not increased above those of any other woman of your age. In the unusual circumstance of the affected person having the rare translocation type of Down syndrome, the parents and other normal family members may have a chromosome rearrangement which increases their risk. It is likely that the parents of the affected person will know if this is the case.

I am young but am very worried about a fetal abnormality. May I have an amniocentesis or CVS?

It is important if you are in this situation that you look closely at why you wish to have the test done and what you would do if the test did show an abnormality. You will need to enquire whether amniocentesis is available to people like yourself. Some centres have limited resources and offer these relatively expensive tests only to couples who fit within certain guidelines, although prenatal testing ideally should be available to all informed couples who request it.

Early in pregnancy I drank too much alcohol/took drugs/had an X-ray/had a severe illness; should I have an amniocentesis or CVS?

None of these external factors increases your chance of having a baby with a chromosomal abnormality. It may be appropriate with some of them to have a careful ultrasound at 18 to 20 weeks, but amniocentesis and CVS do not test for damage caused by any of these substances.

Who makes the decision as to whether amniocentesis or CVS is best for me?

The decision is yours. In this book we have attempted to provide information to allow you to make your own decision. Chapters 6 and 7, which detail the differences between the two tests, should help you decide which is most suited to your situation. Your obstetrician, plus local counselling services, are also available to help you.

Amniocentesis

Amniocentesis (pronounced amneo-sen-tee-sis) was the first test used to check for chromosome disorders in the fetus. Only since the late 1970s and early 1980s has its use become widespread; it is still the most common method used to test fetal chromosomes. This chapter provides detailed information about the procedure, the indications for its use, and the risks involved.

Amniocentesis involves the withdrawal of a sample of fluid from around the developing fetus. A needle is passed through the skin of the pregnant woman, the wall of the uterus, and into the sac containing the amniotic fluid (see figure 6.1). This test can be carried out at any stage of pregnancy, although it is most commonly done at around 15 to 17 weeks.

DEVELOPMENT OF THE TEST

Amniocentesis was the first test introduced in which a needle was used to invade the environment of the developing fetus. It was first carried out in the 1930s to inject dye into the uterus to help outline the fetus on X-ray. By the 1950s it was also used for testing a fetus when its blood group was incompatible with that of the pregnant woman. Amniocentesis to test fetuses for genetic disease was first performed in 1967, and its use has escalated ever since. You can see, therefore, that it is only relatively recently that fetuses have been tested before birth and even more recently that the tests have been in widespread use.

Unlike other tests we will be discussing, amniocentesis was introduced before ultrasound was widely used. Without the benefit of ultrasound to help the doctor accurately place the needle, the method had a risk of 0.6 in 100 of causing a miscarriage. With the widespread use of ultrasound, many studies now show this risk to be even lower.

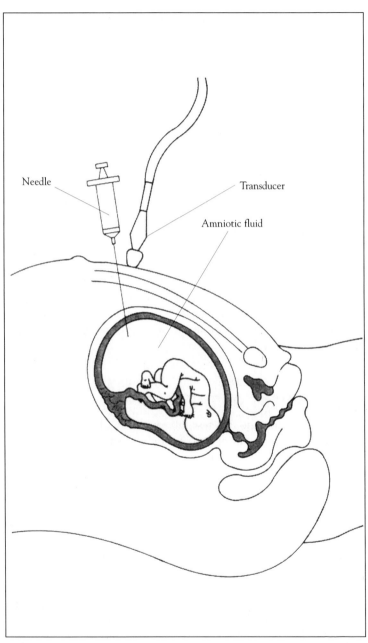

Figure 6.1 Amniocentesis: ultrasound is used to guide the needle into a pocket of fluid.

WHY HAVE AN AMNIOCENTESIS?

In general these tests are offered only to pregnant women who are at increased risk of producing a baby with a very specific abnormality, such as Down syndrome. Amniocentesis is not regarded as a routine test available to every pregnant woman who wants to have all possible checks done on the fetus. This is because there is a small risk involved and because of the associated expense. For most young pregnant women the chance of having a baby with Down syndrome or other chromosome disorders is so low that the tests are considered to be unnecessarily risky. If these tests could pick up all abnormalities the situation might be different, but they can detect only specific abnormalities such as chromosomal defects. There are a host of rare genetic diseases that can be diagnosed by analysing the amniotic fluid, but most of these are only looked for if the couple has previously had a child with this type of disease.

The two most common reasons for undertaking amniocentesis are to check the chromosomes and to look for spina bifida. In most centres older women, usually those 35 years and above, depending on local recommendations, are offered the option of amniocentesis or CVS. By this age the risk of miscarriage from the procedure is similar to that of having a baby with Down syndrome. In many ways, this is an artificial comparison because risks are perceived differently by different women, depending on their attitudes towards disabilities and their childbearing histories. Most Western countries now offer testing to those 35 and above, and sometimes to even younger women. Increasingly, however, all pregnant women are being offered a blood test at 16 weeks: hormones released from the placenta are tested (see chapter 8) and if these show there is a higher than usual risk of Down syndrome, then amniocentesis is offered regardless of the pregnant woman's age.

Amniocentesis can be used to diagnose spina bifida, by measuring the alpha-fetoprotein (AFP) in the amniotic fluid. This is a cheap and easy test, so usually it is routinely carried out on the amniotic sample, even for those at low risk. Spina bifida is one of the few abnormalities which can be tested for by amniocentesis, but not by CVS.

While most amniocenteses are carried out to look for genetic disease, occasionally it is done later in pregnancy for other reasons. These will be discussed in chapter 11, and include testing a fetus whose blood group is incompatible with that of the pregnant woman.

TIMING OF THE TEST

The usual time for performing amniocentesis is between 15 and 17 weeks. While women are keen to get the result as early as possible, studies on the risks when the technique is applied at an earlier stage of pregnancy, such as 10 to 14 weeks, are not yet complete. There was formerly another reason for preferring a later test. At 10 weeks there is only about 30 ml of amniotic fluid in the uterus, which is smaller than the amount of water one can fit into a medicine glass, but by 16 weeks about 200 ml is present, or six to seven times as much. This made it a much easier prospect for the doctor to place the needle into the fluid, and allowed a smaller proportion of the total volume to be taken. Now, with the aid of ultrasound, a needle can be put into the smallest volume of fluid. However, amniocentesis is usually still carried out at the traditional time, and this will be the case until safety studies regarding the risk of 'early' amniocentesis are completed.

It is possible to do the test later than 17 weeks, but the laboratory may take up to three weeks, and occasionally longer, to process it, which means the result comes back very late in pregnancy. Nobody wants to wait longer than necessary to obtain the results. Sometimes it is unavoidable because a pregnant woman does not attend her doctor early in pregnancy, or because the pregnancy is further advanced than expected. If you are unfortunate enough to have an abnormality detected on the amniocentesis, and you want to have the pregnancy terminated, this should be done as early as possible both for emotional and medical reasons. The latest time an abortion can be performed depends on local laws and can be as early as 20 weeks or as late as 24 weeks, depending on where you live. If the fetus has a severe abnormality, which gives it no prospect of survival, an abortion can usually be obtained at any stage.

TERMINATION OF PREGNANCY

From a medical viewpoint, abortion can now be carried out safely at any time of pregnancy. Local laws, however, restrict the stage at which it may be performed. One of the major disadvantages of amniocentesis is that if you choose to have an abortion following abnormal results, the pregnancy will have advanced to 17 to 20 weeks, when it is usually necessary to induce labour. While complications are uncommon at any time, the risks are slightly higher at this late stage.

Uterine contractions are initiated by a substance called prostaglandin, which may be injected into the amniotic fluid, or up through the cervix around the membranes, or simply placed in the vagina. It generally takes 12 to 24 hours until delivery, although most of this time is spent waiting for contractions to start. During labour, pain relief can be achieved if necessary with Pethidine or an epidural anaesthetic. An alternative method is called dilatation and evacuation (D & E). This is performed under anaesthesia and involves dilating the cervix and removing the pregnancy with forceps, so the woman is not required to go through labour.

Even early in pregnancy it is a terribly difficult decision to have an abortion for a very much wanted baby, even though it has been shown to have a major abnormality. If, however, the decision must be made at 20 weeks, and you are already feeling movements, then it is even harder (see chapter 10 for a fuller discussion of this issue). There can be no denying that termination is likely to produce a very painful grief reaction. Women in this situation need plenty of family support and should be offered counselling.

PREPARATION FOR AMNIOCENTESIS

You are likely to feel apprehensive and nervous prior to your amniocentesis, particularly if it is your first one. We hope to alleviate some of that fear by explaining the procedure and emphasizing that most women do not find it painful. It is an exciting experience seeing your unborn baby on the ultrasound screen with all its human features. If you are able to relax enough to watch the TV monitor during the test you may find it fascinating. Many women find it helpful for their partner or a friend to attend amniocentesis with them. Your partner can watch the ultrasound scan and provide moral support. If you both wish him to stay and watch the amniocentesis there is no reason why he should not do so.

You do not need to have any special preparation for amniocentesis. Your doctor may suggest you have an ultrasound examination sometime in the weeks before the amniocentesis if there is any doubt about how advanced your pregnancy is. In the past, women were required to have a full bladder for the ultrasound examination prior to amniocentesis. This is now no longer necessary, although your doctor might ask you to have some urine in your bladder. The ultrasound examination is done in the normal way, followed immediately by the amniocentesis, without you having to move from the examination couch. There is no need to empty your bladder before amniocentesis.

You should know your blood group before amniocentesis. Any procedure that involves passing a needle into the uterus can result in some blood cells from the fetus crossing into the circulation of the pregnant woman. If you are one of the 15 per cent of people who have Rhesus negative blood, the fetal cells may cause you to develop antibodies so that your circulation is cleared of the 'foreign' cells. These antibodies in turn cross the placenta and, particularly in subsequent pregnancies, the level of antibody may rise and destroy enough of the red cells in the fetal circulation to cause it to become anaemic. This is called Rhesus (Rh) disease. To prevent a Rhesus negative pregnant woman making these antibodies, an injection of anti-D may be given to destroy the fetal red blood cells. Usually a blood test is taken before the anti-D injection is given, to ensure there are not already antibodies present. There has been a worldwide shortage of anti-D. This has made it necessary for some countries, including Australia, to import the product.

Rhesus disease is such an uncommon complication of amniocentesis that anti-D is usually recommended only if the needle has to pass through the placenta.

TEST PROCEDURE

An area on the abdomen is prepared by cleansing the skin with antiseptic solution. A local anaesthetic would normally be available if you wish to have it. The ultrasound transducer is placed on the skin and moved around until an area is found where the needle can be inserted straight into the amniotic fluid without making contact with the fetus or placenta (see figure 6.2). The needle is plunged rapidly through the skin, down to the appropriate depth (see figure 6.3).

The doctor watches the needle on the ultrasound screen from the moment it enters the skin until it is withdrawn, and so is able to adjust its position to avoid the fetus if it comes near. There are two ways of guiding the needle. The first, shown in figure 6.2, involves passing the needle through a frame attached to the side of the ultrasound transducer. Those who use this method usually use the software of the ultrasound equipment to plot a dotted line down the screen and this is the course the needle will follow. It is then a fairly simple matter to line up the most readily available pool of

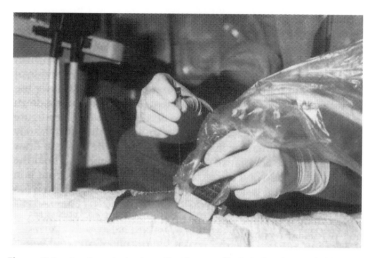

Figure 6.2 Amniocentesis: here the fine needle is being inserted through a frame to guide it to the correct place. The ultrasound transducer is in a sterile plastic bag.

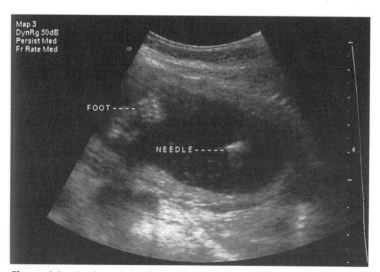

Figure. 6.3 Amniocentesis: the needle tip (Ne) is visible as the doctor guides it with the aid of ultrasound. The foot had to be watched carefully to ensure that it stayed away from the needle.

amniotic fluid and place the needle into it to draw off the fluid. The alternative or 'freehand' technique is to hold the needle in one hand and the ultrasound transducer away from it in the other hand and watch the needle from a distance. Research has demonstrated no difference in the safety of the two techniques. The critical thing is that the operator be confident and experienced at whichever technique is used.

Surprisingly, it is unusual to have to pass the needle through the placenta to get into the amniotic fluid. Even when the placenta is on the front (or anterior) wall of the uterus it rarely covers the entire wall; a 'placenta-free' space is usually available somewhere. Occasionally there is no 'placenta-free' area, and in this case the doctor would find a thin area of placenta and pass the needle accurately through it. Many doctors try to find a site high up in the uterus as this might help minimize the chance of fluid leakage after the test.

Once the needle is in the appropriate place a syringe is attached. The first 1 or 2 ml are usually discarded as they are more likely to contain cells collected from the pregnant woman's tissues. About 15 ml of fluid is withdrawn, the needle is removed and the heartbeat of the fetus rechecked. If the test is carried out as described, there is virtually never any irregularity of the heartbeat afterwards.

The important point about the amniocentesis itself is that the doctor needs to be experienced in performing the technique under ultrasound guidance. It is reasonable to expect your doctor to be doing at least 50 amniocenteses per year.

WILL THE TEST HURT?

Amniocentesis performed by an experienced doctor does not usually cause you more than mild discomfort. To many people it is no more painful than a blood test. When patients at a Melbourne clinic were asked to fill out a questionnaire after amniocentesis, 83 per cent said that the test was less painful than they had expected. Some 86 per cent said it caused no or only mild discomfort, while 14 per cent said it had caused some pain. Because most women dread the procedure, they are almost universally surprised that a needle can be passed into the uterus with minimal discomfort.

> I had read enough about amniocentesis to think that it would be awful. My husband came along and we had both built up a lot of apprehension. But I was lucky. The gynaecologist was terrific, probably the best around. It was definitely uncomfortable seeing the

needle go into my abdomen, but it was not painful. I was distracted by the procedure, so the ultrasound examination of the fetus had little impact. We had been ambivalent about having children, but my husband fell in love with our son when he saw him on the ultrasound screen.

For most women amniocentesis is a psychologically stressful experience, a focus for all their fears about abnormalities. As for physical pain, experiences vary. Apart from the skin and peritoneum, the needle passes through layers such as muscle, fatty tissue and the uterus, which have few pain fibres. A very fine needle is used, usually 22 gauge, which minimizes the risk and causes no distress to most women.

A local anaesthetic can be used to desensitize the skin, although most doctors do not encourage this. This is not just for the doctor's convenience, but rather because the procedure is actually less painful if you do *not* have the local anaesthetic. The solution of local anaesthetic requires an injection which stings as it goes in, and then a second needle must be inserted for amniocentesis. Experienced operators are able to pass the needle into the amniotic fluid on the first attempt on nearly every occasion. Most people will feel that the pain of the anaesthetic injection is worse than the passage of the needle without it. Women who are very anxious about the procedure can benefit from using nitrous oxide (the 'laughing gas' used in labour).

AFTER THE TEST

In previous years, women were asked to stay in hospital after the test and have strict bed rest, but this is no longer considered necessary. After you have had the test it will probably be suggested that you sit down and wait for a short time before you depart. You will be quite capable of driving yourself home. Many women feel emotionally drained afterwards as they have been psychologically preparing for the test for some time and appreciate having somebody to accompany them home. It is a good idea to relax at home for the rest of the day, although there should be no reason to go to bed. Occasionally the needle may puncture a small blood vessel under your skin resulting in a bruise and minor discomfort. In general, most doctors would recommend a return to normal activities after the day of the test and for the remainder of the pregnancy.

RISKS TO THE FETUS

The most drastic complication and the one most universally feared is a miscarriage due to the amniocentesis. There have been many studies assessing the risks of the procedure, and the most constant finding, one shown by virtually all, is that there is an increased risk of miscarriage. Putting a precise figure on that risk is more difficult. Different operators use different techniques, which may have different complication rates. It is also difficult to tell if a pregnancy loss after amniocentesis is because of the procedure or whether it would have occurred anyway. It is likely that a miscarriage the day after was due to the test and one four weeks later was not, but it is impossible to be sure. Figures are published that report the loss rates of major centres around the world. These estimate that amniocentesis increases the risk of miscarriage by about 0.5 per cent.

About 0.7 per cent of pregnancies that appear normal on ultrasound at 16 weeks will subsequently miscarry, if amniocentesis is not performed. This is called the 'background' rate. Unfortunately this background rate is not a precise figure. To find out how many pregnancies miscarry after amniocentesis, the background rate is subtracted from the total number that miscarry. This gives an approximate rate of miscarriage due to the test, which should be available information for interested couples.

One of the things you may be most fearful of is that the needle may penetrate the fetus. Earlier studies showed that between 1 and 3 per cent of babies showed evidence after birth of being touched by the needle. Most cases involved dimples or skin scars. These mostly occurred prior to the use of modern ultrasound machines to monitor the test. As the needle will be constantly watched with ultrasound on the television monitor, this can nearly always be avoided. Even if the fetus comes near, the needle can be moved to keep out of its way. If the needle did touch the fetus it would do no more damage than having a needle passed into the same place on your body. Fetuses have been tranfused before birth, with needles being passed into their legs and body at least a dozen times, without a single mark being visible on the skin after birth.

One large study suggested there was an increased chance of the baby being born with club feet or dislocated hips after amniocentesis. Other studies have not confirmed this. A group of children with these abnormalities was looked at, and amniocentesis was not shown to be a cause. It is unlikely, therefore, that the risk of these postural abnormalities is increased by the test.

Several studies have suggested there is a slight increase of about 0.6 per cent in the risk of breathing disorders immediately after birth, particularly in babies born between 34 and 37 weeks. The reason for this increase is unknown, and it has not been proved to be a complication of amniocenteis. One suggestion is that it is related to the volume of fluid aspirated and that a maximum of 17 ml should be removed.

OTHER COMPLICATIONS

Complications rarely occur after the test. You may feel tired due to the anxiety associated with the procedure and its implications. Studies of many patients suggest that amniotic fluid may leak from the vagina in about 1 per cent of amniocenteses, presumably leaking through a hole in the membranes. If this happened there would be a small gush of clear fluid from the vagina, usually in the few days immediately after the test. When this occurs at other times the outlook is very poor, but after amniocentesis the leak usually lasts only a short time or is a single gush. The fluid loss usually settles rapidly and the pregnancy continues normally. Only rarely does the fluid loss continue.

If you have abdominal pain or if you lose water or blood through the vagina you should report it to your doctor — usually bed rest will be recommended. If this did happen you would notice without specifically watching for it. Any such symptoms usually settle. It does not necessarily mean you will miscarry.

The risks of the test to the pregnant woman are extremely low. Theoretically passing a 'foreign body', the needle, into the uterus could cause infection, but this has rarely been reported. One study showed that generalized infection occurred in only one of 7579 patients.

As mentioned earlier in this chapter, the risk of Rhesus negative women developing antibodies after amniocentesis is very low, and anti-D is not usually administered unless the needle passes through the placenta.

Minimizing the Complications

If a needle is passed straight into the amniotic fluid there is very rarely blood staining — one series of 500 women was tested without a single specimen being blood-stained. Blood staining tends to occur if there are technical difficulties during amniocentesis. It has been suggested that if this happens there is a two- or three-fold increase in the risk of miscarriage, but even then the risk is quite low. Blood-stained amniotic fluid should not be confused with brown fluid. This is not due to the amniocentesis, but usually to old blood which accumulated at the time of an earlier threatened miscarriage. When the amniotic fluid is brown there might be a slight increase in the risk of miscarriage, not because of the amniocentesis but because of the earlier bleeding.

Studies have shown that two insertions of the needle are required in 2 to 3 per cent of amniocenteses. It has been suggested that multiple needle insertions increase the miscarriage rate following the test, the risk increasing with each needle pass. Some studies have also suggested an increased risk if the needle must pass through the placenta, although others have found no such increase. One would expect that the increased risk would depend on how thick a portion of the placenta was traversed. If care is taken to pass through a thin portion, any risk increase is likely to be minimal.

PROCESSING THE SPECIMEN

The specimen is sent to a laboratory where it is processed for analysis. It is put into a centrifuge, which spins all the cells to the bottom of the flask. Some of the fluid is taken off the top to analyse for alpha-fetoprotein, the test for spina bifida. The cells at the bottom of the flask are placed into a culture dish or bottle with culture medium containing antibiotics. This is then placed into an incubator and the cells allowed to grow. These cells come from the fetal skin, connective tissue, lining of respiratory, alimentary and urinary tracts and from the amniotic membranes.

The growth can take anything from a few days to occasionally as long as four weeks. When adequate numbers of colonies or cells have grown, the specimen is taken out of the incubator and carefully examined. At least fifteen cells are usually analysed. The chromosomes are counted to ensure that there are 46, and they are individually examined to make sure the structure or banding of each appears normal. This is a lengthy process requiring highly skilled personnel. A photograph is taken of the chromosomes from one or two cells. Each chromosome is then cut out, paired with its opposite member and placed in numerical sequence.

WAITING FOR THE RESULTS

The time taken for you to receive the results can be anything from one to four weeks, or sometimes longer. These times vary because laboratory techniques differ. But even within one laboratory reporting times vary with the speed of growth of the cells and the workload. The wait for the result is likely to be the most difficult part of the test for you. No matter how small the chance of the results being abnormal, your attention is likely to be focused on the result. The main reason that CVS has become so popular is that results are available much earlier (see chapter 7).

TEST FAILURE

Amniocentesis has now been refined to such a stage that once you have decided to have the test you can be almost sure it will be successful. However, even in the most experienced hands a test may fail. About 1 per cent of women require a repeat test, either because fluid is not obtained or because of problems with the laboratory culture. Technical difficulties are uncommon during an amniocentesis, except in the rare situation where there is very little fluid around the fetus. Occasionally, the laboratory may receive a good specimen, but for some inexplicable reason none of the cells grow and so cannot be analysed. One reason for failed growth is that bacteria somehow get into the specimen. The laboratory also has difficulty if the specimen is very blood-stained, a rare occurrence using the technique described.

AMNIOCENTESIS IN MULTIPLE PREGNANCIES

If you have a twin pregnancy it is more likely that the fetuses will be non-identical, particularly if you are over 35. Non-identical twins have a risk of an abnormality in *each* fetus similar to that of a single fetus. Therefore, overall you have about double the risk of having a fetus with an abnormality compared to someone with a single fetus. If you have triplets the risk increases threefold, and so on. Amniocentesis is performed for the same reasons as a single pregnancy, such the age of the pregnant woman. Since two insertions of the needle are necessary with twins, there is likely to be an increased risk. Results vary, but reports suggest the risk of miscarriage is around 1 per cent.

If amniocentesis is performed using the technique discussed in this chapter, there is usually no problem sampling the fluid in the sac around each of the fetuses to test them individually. The doctor carefully searches for the membrane between the two fetuses and makes sure that fluid is taken from each sac in turn, usually by passing a needle through the skin at two separate sites. After taking the first specimen, a dye may be injected into the fluid, to ensure it is not sampled again. Many doctors believe this dye is no longer necessary.

If you plan to have an amniocentesis with a multiple pregnancy, it is worth considering what options would be available if a serious abnormality was found. Any abnormality would usually affect just one fetus, with the other(s) being normal. In this situation three options would be available. First, you could continue the pregnancy knowing one fetus is abnormal, but being prepared to accept that outcome. Second, the pregnancy could be terminated, both the normal and the abnormal fetuses being aborted together. Finally, there is the option known as selective reduction, which involves injecting into the heart of the abnormal fetus a solution of a potassium salt, causing it to die instantly. The risk to the surviving fetuses appears to be low. The dead fetus stays in the uterus and is delivered at the end of the pregnancy, without affecting the growth or well-being of the live fetus(es).

Selective reduction would not be carried out if it appeared that the fetuses were monozygous (that is, come from one egg with one placenta), because then there could be a mixing of the circulation of the fetuses at the placenta, in which case the death of one could affect the surviving identical twin. Fortunately, most twin pregnancies in which one of the fetuses is abnormal are dizygous (that is, come from two eggs). If you would plan to accept option one, continuing with the pregnancy, then you might consider not having amniocentesis. Most opt for the injection rather than aborting the normal fetus as well.

Questions

How long does the needle stay inside me?
The time taken between insertion of the needle through the skin and removing it after withdrawing the fluid is around 30 seconds. Once the needle is placed in the fluid it does not have to be moved, so it does not hurt at all as the fluid is being withdrawn.

You will have no 'pulling' inside and no other feelings as the fluid is removed from your uterus.

Can my cells grow in the laboratory instead of those of the fetus?
This is called 'contamination' of the specimen with your cells. As the methods described in this chapter are so reliable it is now very rare indeed for contamination to occur.

If miscarriage occurred, when would it happen?
Unfortunately there is no simple answer to this question. There is no way of telling whether a miscarriage after amniocentesis is due to the amniocentesis or would have occurred anyway. Since miscarriages can occur at any stage in pregnancy, whether or not you have an amniocentesis, there is no time that you can say you are 'totally safe'. It is presumed in general that miscarriages in the few weeks after amniocentesis are more likely to be due to the test than those that occur much later. The important thing to remember is that this is a low-risk technique and it is rare to miscarry as a result of it.

Why is the fluid yellow?
When red blood cells are broken down in the body a yellow substance called bilirubin is produced. The bilirubin tends to accumulate in the amniotic fluid in early pregnancy and gives it the yellow colour, which is quite normal. As pregnancy advances the fluid tends to become clearer.

How do you make sure the needle will not touch the fetus?
At amniocentesis a pool of amniotic fluid is taken away from the fetus. While theoretically the doctor could go off course and touch the fetus, or alternatively the fetus could move into the path of the needle, as long as the doctor watches the needle with ultrasound, it is usually easily avoided. Even if the fetus did come in contact with the needle, it would not be harmed. Indeed, as we will see in chapter 11, the baby is sometimes pricked by the needle deliberately for testing or treatment.

How much fluid does the doctor take?
Usually about 15 ml, which is less than 10 per cent of the amount of fluid present at 16 weeks.

How long does it take for the fluid to be replaced?
The fetus continuously produces and removes the fluid around itself. By the end of pregnancy more than a litre of amniotic fluid

is produced daily and the same amount removed. It is hard to tell how long it takes for the total amount of fluid present to return to what it was before the amniocentesis, but it is presumably over the course of several days.

Won't the fluid leak out the hole in my skin?

The needle used is so fine that the hole closes off immediately and fluid does not come out through the skin afterwards.

I have a brother or sister with spina bifida. Should I have an amniocentesis?

Usually it is not recommended. Your unborn baby has approximately a 0.5 per cent risk of having spina bifida, with an equal risk of anencephaly. Ultrasound will detect all cases of anencephaly after 13 weeks and approximately 95 per cent of spina bifida at 18 weeks. If you have a normal ultrasound at 18 weeks, then the chance of the fetus having spina bifida is only about one in 2000. Amniocentesis would be unnecessarily risky by comparison. As an added precaution an AFP test on your blood may be suggested (see chapter 8).

Can amniocentesis tell the sex of the fetus?

Analysis of the chromosomes automatically indicates the sex. Your obstetrician can tell you the sex if you wish to know.

Is it true that I must have an amniocentesis if I'm over thirty-seven?

Amniocentesis is an option available to couples who are seeking prenatal diagnosis. There is never any compulsion to have the test. You are welcome to seek medical advice, but ultimately you are free to make your own decision.

Earlier Testing with CVS

Chorionic villus sampling (CVS) was introduced in the mid 1980s primarily as a method of testing fetal chromosomes. Its popularity rests on the fact that it can be carried out much earlier than amniocentesis. This chapter explains what to expect from a CVS procedure, and aims to help you understand and assess its benefits and risks.

You may not have heard of chorionic villus sampling (usually abbreviated to CVS) because it is much newer than amniocentesis. It is, however, widely available. Many centres have found a remarkably rapid swing away from amniocentesis to CVS, the great attraction being that the results are available very much earlier in pregnancy. There is, however, considered to be a greater risk of miscarriage with CVS, although only slightly higher than amniocentesis when performed by an experienced operator.

Chorionic (pronounced ko-re-on-ik) villus sampling is a test involving the passage of a needle or cannula into the placenta in order to withdraw a few small fragments of the tissue into a syringe. It is called 'chorionic' because the chorion is the name for the placenta in the very early stages of pregnancy. The name 'villus' is derived from the microscopic appearance of the chorionic surface — large numbers of finger-like structures or 'villi' projecting outwards towards the lining of the uterus. Chorionic villus sampling is occasionally called 'placental biopsy' or 'placentocentesis'.

DEVELOPMENT OF THE TEST

CVS was first used in Denmark in 1968, but was abandoned because it caused too many miscarriages. It was, however, quickly taken up by the Chinese who used CVS to determine the sex of fetuses early in pregnancy to ensure that male children were born. It was first used to test for abnormalities in the USSR in 1982 and then subsequently in Europe. Initially, all specimens were taken by passing a cannula through the vagina and the cervix up into the uterus. But in 1984 the first successful attempts were made using the alternative approach whereby a needle is passed through the abdominal wall and uterus and then into the placenta.

When CVS was first used, many methods of obtaining placental tissue were tried. Success rates with these different methods varied but commonly they caused a very high miscarriage rate. As techniques were refined only those methods with a low miscarriage rate were used widely in clinical practice. Today all biopsies are taken under the guidance of ultrasound. In experienced hands, CVS is now believed to increase the miscarriage rate by a maximum of 1 per cent.

WHY HAVE A CVS?

CVS and amniocentesis are offered to pregnant women who are at increased risk of carrying a fetus with specific abnormalities. They are not general tests to see if the fetus is normal. While there are a host of genetic diseases that can be tested for by analysing chorionic villi, most of the diseases are very rare and would only be looked for if there was a family history of a disorder which could be passed onto a child. The only common reason for testing chorionic villi is to check the chromosomes. The reasons for performing CVS were discussed in detail in Chapter 5. By far the most common reason is because the pregnant woman is in her late thirties or forties and therefore is at greater risk of having a Down syndrome baby. The second most common reason is because a woman has previously had a baby with a chromosomal abnormality.

If the test is to be performed to check the chromosomes there is a choice of CVS or amniocentesis. While most diseases which can be tested by amniocentesis can also be tested by CVS, there is one important abnormality for which CVS is not applicable — spina bifida.

There are two reasons why this inability to test for spina bifida on CVS is usually unimportant. Spina bifida is a rare condition in most countries and, unlike Down syndrome, its incidence does not increase with the age of the pregnant woman. Therefore most women having a CVS are at low risk of carrying a fetus with spina bifida. In addition, ultrasound is now so good at detecting spina bifida that it will usually be diagnosed if those women who have a CVS also have a scan at 18 weeks.

WHO SHOULD PERFORM THE CVS?

The best test for you depends on expertise in your region. Before making your decision on amniocentesis or on transabdominal or transcervical CVS (see below), you should ask your obstetrician which techniques local experts usually perform. A major US study suggested that doctors need to perform approximately 75 CVS tests in order to learn the technique. Performance improves considerably with experience. Independent follow-up of women who have undergone CVS have shown miscarriage rates as high as 20 per cent. These high rates can be attributed to the inexperience of the operators and highlight the importance of selecting the best expertise available. It has been suggested that skill improves over the first 100 cases of transabdominal CVS and over the first 300 transcervical tests. To maintain expertise at least 50 procedures per year should be performed. The doctor performing the CVS should also be able to tell you how many patients miscarry after the procedure in his or her particular practice. Experienced centres generally quote 1 per cent as the miscarriage rate attributed to CVS. On top of this is the 'background' risk: even without the test about 2.5 per cent of women whose pregnancy appears normal at 10 weeks will miscarry. The background risk increases with the age of the pregnant woman.

WHEN IS THE BEST TIME FOR A CVS?

The usual time to perform CVS is between 10 and 12 weeks, but it can be performed any time after 10 weeks. By 10 weeks the placenta thickens in one area and it is possible to recognize where the fully formed placenta will be situated. This is an easier target for the needle.

If the direct method of chromosome analysis is used, it may provide the chromosome result in a few days. Otherwise, the laboratory needs about two weeks to process the specimen, in which case you will be told the result at 12 weeks. At this time you do not look pregnant and have not felt movements. If you are unfortunate enough to have an abnormality detected and you request an abortion, it is still early enough to dilate the cervix and carry out a simple curettage operation. It takes only a few minutes and usually it is unnecessary to stay overnight in hospital. CVS can also be performed later in pregnancy when it is often called placental biopsy.

PREPARATION FOR CVS

Your doctor may suggest you have an ultrasound examination some time before your CVS if there is any doubt about the age of your pregnancy or if you have had some complication such as bleeding. In addition, if a transcervical CVS is planned a swab may be taken from your cervix to look for bacterial infection to avoid the possibility of infection being introduced into the uterus at the time of CVS. Such an infection will usually be treated with antibiotics first or alternatively a transabdominal CVS performed instead.

You do not need to have any special preparation on the day of your CVS. The only thing your doctor may ask you to do is to have some urine in your bladder either for the ultrasound or for the CVS, particularly if it is transcervical. The ultrasound is carried out in the usual way, followed immediately by the CVS without you having to move from the examination couch.

The doctor will also want to know your blood group before CVS. This is because some blood cells from the fetus may cross into your own circulation during the procedure. If you are one of the 15 per cent of women who are Rh negative, your body might produce antibodies to these cells which cause problems in subsequent pregnancies. Women with Rh negative blood group will, therefore, be given an 'anti-D' injection to prevent such an occurrence.

HOW IS THE TEST DONE?

There are two commonly used methods of passing a needle into the developing placenta.

(i)   The most widely used method has been to pass a cannula through the cervix and into the uterus to the developing placenta; this is transcervical CVS (figure 7.1).

(ii) The second method is to pass a fine needle through the skin of the abdominal wall, through the uterus and down into the placenta; this is a transabdominal CVS (figure 7.2). From the pregnant woman's point of view, this is very similar to an amniocentesis.

Which method is used depends partly on medical factors (see table 7.1) but above all on the expertise of the operator.

Transcervical CVS

For a transcervical CVS it is necessary for the bladder to be full. Prior to the test the doctor will check that there is an appropriate amount

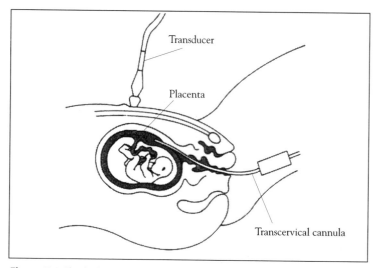

Figure 7.1 Chorionic villus sampling (CVS), using the transcervical method: a cannula is passed up through the cervix then guided into the placenta with ultrasound.

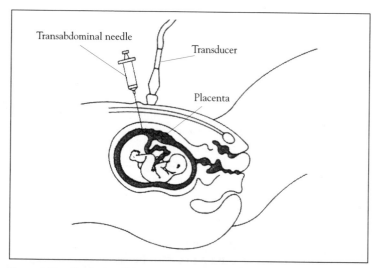

Figure. 7.2 Chorionic villus sampling (CVS), using the transabdominal technique: a needle is passed through the abdomen down into the placenta.

TABLE 7.1 FACTORS INFLUENCING THE CHOICE BETWEEN
TRANSABDOMINAL AND TRANSCERVICAL CVS

	Transcervical	Transabdominal
Access difficult:		
— cervical fibroid	Difficult	No difficulty
— sharply retroverted uterus	May be difficult	May be difficult
— sharply anteverted uterus	May be difficult	No difficulty
Vaginal infection	Avoid	No problem
Risk of test*	Low in experienced hands	Low in experienced hands

*The most important determinant of risk is the experience and expertise of the
doctor performing the test.

of urine in your bladder at the same time as the fetus is scanned. You
will then be asked to lie on your back with your legs lifted and held
apart in stirrups at the foot of the couch. After washing in and around
the vagina with an antiseptic solution the doctor passes a speculum
(a metal or plastic object which holds the walls of the vagina apart)
into the vagina to view the cervix. Having located the cervix, if necessary he or she grasps it with a pair of forceps. This may produce a
pinching sensation.

The specimen is taken by passing a blunt cannula up through the
cervix into the uterus, then advancing it into the developing placental tissue. By placing the ultrasound transducer onto the skin of
your abdominal wall, the doctor is able to watch the cannula as it
passes through the cervix and carefully guide it into the placenta. An
anaesthetic is not used. Any irregularity of the wall of the uterus can
usually be negotiated by careful and gentle manipulation.

The cannula is made of either soft, bendable stainless steel,
which is sterilized between patients, or of a disposable plastic. Most
people feel very little as it is passed into the uterus because even in
pregnancy the neck of the womb is sufficiently open to allow the

passage of this fine cannula. Once the tip of the cannula is in the placenta, suction is applied to the syringe at the other end and the tip of the cannula is moved around within the placenta to obtain tissue. The cannula is then withdrawn, the tissue ejected from the syringe and inspected to see if there is enough. If there are not enough villi in the specimen, the test can be repeated by passing a second cannula through the neck of the womb. Test repetition depends on the experience of the operator and can occur in as few as 7 per cent of cases and as many as 45 per cent. If inadequate material is obtained after two or three attempts, the procedure would usually be rescheduled since by continuing to repeat the test on the same day, there is an increased risk of miscarriage. The pregnancy and the fetal heartbeat are rechecked after the test.

Once the CVS has been completed, your legs are taken out of the stirrups and you lie on the couch for a short time before emptying your bladder. There may be some slight vaginal bleeding. It may be suggested that you sit and relax for a while before going home.

This test is not used if you have an untreated vaginal infection, are unable to accept any vaginal examination, have a fibroid low in the uterus which would be difficult to bypass, or if you present for CVS after 11 or 12 weeks.

Transabdominal CVS

If the transabdominal approach is used most doctors would not ask you to have a full bladder. The ultrasound examination is carried out and instead of placing your legs in stirrups, you remain lying flat on the couch. The doctor then locates the best place to pass the needle through your skin and, if local anaesthetic is to be used, injects it into that site. Most doctors give an anaesthetic, but it is difficult to know how much benefit it provides. It is used to anaesthetize the skin and the layers immediately beneath. It is not used to anaesthetize the layers deep inside the abdomen and if any discomfort occurs with this test, it is usually from these deeper layers. Nitrous oxide (the 'gas' commonly used during labour) is more effective in relieving any pain.

The specimen is taken by passing a needle down through the wall of your abdomen (as shown in figure 7.2) and into the placenta. This needle is carefully guided by watching it with ultrasound. It may be guided by using an attachment at the side of the ultrasound transducer to hold the needle on a predetermined course, which is shown on the screen as a dotted line. An alternative technique is to hold the transducer at a distance from the needle to watch its advance. The best method to use is the one with which the operator is most comfortable.

Once the needle tip is placed through the wall of the uterus and situated in the placental tissue, the sample can be taken. This is usually done by feeding a second needle down the inside of the first and moving it up and down in the placental tissue whilst applying suction with a syringe at the other end. It can also be performed by applying suction to a single needle. The advantage of the two-needle method is that if there is inadequate material the fine needle can be painlessly passed down the inside of the wider bore needle to take a further sample. Depending on the width of the needle, it can take several aspirations to obtain enough material.

When the tissue has been inspected and found to be adequate, the needle is withdrawn. The laboratory likes to receive at least 10 mg for analysis. This amount of tissue is visible to the naked eye and looks like a few flecks floating in the fluid at the bottom of a flask. After the test, the pregnancy and the fetal heartbeat are checked before you leave the room.

Minor variations to the techniques described are used at different centres. A wide variety of needles is used, and indeed fine forceps may be used to take the sample of tissue rather than a needle. There are advantages and disadvantages of each technique, but ultimately the equipment selected comes down to personal preference of the doctor. Even if you decide you would prefer a particular approach it is usually better to have whatever method is offered. If a doctor is asked to change his or her technique the results may not be as good. You would do better to change to a doctor who uses the method you prefer rather than asking your own to change.

WILL THE TEST HURT?

For most women CVS is not a painful test. Whichever method is used it is readily tolerated. In the transcervical test, some people find having a full bladder and their legs in stirrups disturbing. If an instrument is used to grasp the cervix, it might cause discomfort. Usually the passage of the cannula into the placenta is not particularly unpleasant.

If the CVS is transabdominal, it is usually tolerated well. It is little different from an amniocentesis and although a slightly wider needle is used, it is generally associated with little pain. In a survey of 50 women who underwent transabdominal CVS in a Melbourne practice, 90 per cent reported no or only mild pain. The other 10 per cent described the pain as moderate and none reported severe pain. One situation that can cause pain is in the rare case where the uterus is tilted backwards (retroverted) and the placenta inserted in the back wall of the uterus. This makes it more difficult to reach with the needle. Nitrous oxide may be used to ensure that the procedure is pain free, although usually only local anaesthetic is offered. Two women who have undergone CVS give their impressions of the procedure:

I had another surprise pregnancy and this time I chose a CVS. It would only involve a curette rather than going through labour if a termination was necessary. From my reading, the risks weren't that much greater than amniocentesis. The procedure amazed me. The needle went through my abdomen, into the uterus and was dipped in and out. This had to be done four or five times, but it was not painful. I was quite philosophical about it. The pregnancy was unexpected and if it wasn't to be, then I would cope with that when the time came.

When I found out I was pregnant, I went to the gynaecologist quickly because I wanted to have a CVS. I had heard it was the same procedure as amniocentesis but that it was done earlier at 10 weeks. I found the risk of miscarriage of 1 per cent quite acceptable. Initially, my husband was against the test because he didn't want me to terminate the pregnancy if the baby was found to have Down syndrome. When I explained how a disabled child would reduce the amount of attention we could show our daughter, he mellowed. The actual test was frightening but straightforward. The needle only had to go in once and there was no pain, just discomfort. It was wonderful having test results back so early because it relieved all the pressures.

In the survey of 50 women who had transabdominal CVS, 17 (34 per cent) also developed abdominal discomfort after the test. This was described as mild by 13, moderate by three, and severe by one. The one woman with severe pain had a similarly severe reaction to having a blood test. The pain began between one and 15 minutes after the CVS and lasted between two and 20 minutes. It was probably due to uterine contractions, which subsided in all cases.

THE RISK OF COMPLICATIONS

The thought of passing a needle into the placenta with its very rich blood supply is initially frightening. Anybody who has seen the large blood vessels leading to the placenta would expect such a test to cause severe bleeding. Clinical trials have shown that this rarely happens.

As the needle does not enter the amniotic sac or pass near the fetus there is very little chance of hurting the fetus itself. The main risk is of miscarriage due to the test, and experienced doctors who have performed large numbers of CVS tests would usually quote it as a maximum of 1 per cent.

Complications of any procedure may be immediate or occur some time later. Significant immediate complications other than pain and failure to obtain a specimen are uncommon. It is possible to rupture the pregnancy sac at the time of the test, but this is rare with an experienced operator. If this happens with a transcervical CVS the pregnancy may miscarry because the cannula leaves such a large hole. If, on the other hand, it happens at transabdominal CVS it may not cause any complication as the needle is much finer. Another complication is the formation of a clot at the site from which the specimen was taken. Again this is rare and if it occurs it will usually resolve without any ill effect.

The most important delayed complication is miscarriage. This will not differ from miscarriage unrelated to CVS — both begin with bleeding. It is difficult to know the exact risk of CVS causing a miscarriage. It is estimated that if a fetus is alive at 10 weeks there is a chance of about 2.5 per cent that it will miscarry anyway without being tested. The chance of miscarriage unrelated to CVS increases with the age of the pregnant woman. If she is 37 years or more then the figure rises.

To determine the risk of miscarriage due to CVS a study would need to be carried out in which women are randomly assigned to CVS or no test (not even amniocentesis later) and the miscarriage rates compared. This type of study is impossible as couples wish to have the right to choose to have a test. Two studies, one from Canada and one from the USA, compared the miscarriage rate after transcervical CVS to that after amniocentesis. They found that CVS caused 0.6 and 0.8 per cent more miscarriages than amniocentesis respectively. Both of these studies were carried out at multiple centres, and some units produced better and some worse results than this — emphasizing the point that the risks depend on who performs the test.

A subsequent USA study by the same group showed that with continued experience the risks became close to those associated with amniocentesis. Results of transabdominal CVS are similar — the most important factor with both is the experience of the operator.

Significant complications other than miscarriages are rare following CVS. Some slight bleeding is common after transcervical CVS, but is rare after transabdominal. The bleeding usually settles within a few days. CVS should not damage the placenta. If the placenta is examined following CVS it is difficult to find any sign that the test was performed. There is no evidence of long-term damage to the placenta — fetuses that have had CVS grow just as well as those that have not had the test.

There are reported cases of severe infection following transcervical CVS resulting in miscarriage and severe illness in the pregnant woman. Because of this, transcervical CVS is not carried out if there is untreated infection in the cervix. It is a very rare complication — no cases occurred in the 2235 women who underwent transcervical CVS in the USA study quoted above.

It has been suggested that 'amputation'-type defects of the arms and legs can follow CVS. The reports included babies born with missing fingers, toes, or lower parts of the arm or leg. Although this initially caused a major scare, subsequent studies from experienced units were unable to find this association. After studying the available information a group, which included the World Health Organisation, concluded that 'present evidence of an increased incidence of limb reduction defects is consistent with an association of very early sampling (at or before 8 menstrual weeks) with some fetal limb abnormalities. There is no evidence to suggest an increased risk of congential malformation when the CVS is performed after the 8th completed menstrual week.'

The groups that reported these abnormalities after CVS were inexperienced, and tended to perform CVS very early in the pregnancy, that is, before 9 weeks. CVS should not be performed before 9 weeks and it should be performed by an experienced operator; when performed under these conditions there is no known increased risk of limb abnormalities.

WHAT TO EXPECT AFTER THE TEST

After you have had the test it will probably be suggested that you wait for a short time before you go home. You will be quite capable of driving yourself home. However, many women feel emotionally drained afterwards as they have been psychologically preparing for the test for some time, and appreciate having someone to accompany them. It is probably a good idea to relax at home for the rest of the day, although there should be no reason to go to bed. While doctors may make slightly differing recommendations, the principles are that after any test in which a needle is passed into the uterus it is recommended that you rest at least the remainder of the day. In general, most doctors would recommend no restriction of activities the following day or for the rest of the pregnancy.

Some bleeding from the vagina is very common after a transcervical CVS. This bleeding often arises from the lower part of the uterus away from the pregnancy, either from the trauma to the uterus itself or from where the cervix was grasped. It usually settles very quickly but may be followed by some brown staining for a day or two as the last of the blood drains away.

Bleeding is rare after transabdominal CVS as the lower part of the uterus has not been interfered with. As discussed earlier, some women have discomfort in the lower abdomen for a short time after the test. This nearly always settles very quickly and is not associated with a risk of miscarriage or damage to the developing pregnancy.

It is rare to have any other problems after a CVS. If you do have any other symptoms, such as continued bleeding, pain or loss of fluid, it is important that you contact your obstetrician. Even if you are unlucky enough to have any of these symptoms, they are likely to settle and your pregnancy continue unaffected.

If you do miscarry after the test, there is no way of telling whether the test was responsible as the symptoms are identical to those of any other miscarriage. The first thing you would notice is bleeding. Your doctor may then suggest you have an ultrasound examination to check whether the fetus is still alive. If it is alive then you should rest in bed until the bleeding stops. If you do miscarry it is not possible to predict when it will happen. Miscarriage can occur at any time during the pregnancy, whether you have a test or not. Even one within two weeks of testing could be a 'natural miscarriage' as these also tend to occur earlier rather than later in the pregnancy.

PROCESSING OF THE SPECIMEN

The chorionic tissue is placed in a dish or flask containing a special fluid. It is examined either with a low-power microscope or with the naked eye to see if there is adequate material. The aim is to obtain a minimum of 10 mg of villi from the placenta for processing. Where possible, it is preferable that this is taken immediately to the laboratory.

In the laboratory the chorionic villi are carefully dissected to remove any decidual cells, that is, those from the pregnant woman, which line the uterus and are often also aspirated during CVS. Either or both of the following methods are then used:

(i)   the chromosomes are looked at either without culturing or by culturing for a short period of up to 24 hours.

(ii) the specimen is cultured for one week or more prior to processing. The cells are taken from the incubator (harvested) when adequate numbers of colonies of cells have grown.

When CVS initially became available the first method was used, which provided virtually immediate results. It was discovered, however, that occasionally the chromosome result was different from that of the fetus. Many laboratories now use this method, and follow up with the long-term method to confirm the results. Others use only one of the two methods. In the first method, the lining cells of the villi of the placenta (the cytotrophoblastic cells) are analysed while in the long-term method the core of the villi (the mesenchymal cells) are analysed. For complex reasons associated with the early development of these two tissues, the chromosomes can occasionally differ.

WAITING FOR THE RESULTS

Laboratories that use the long-term culture will usually provide a final result within 10 to 14 days. If the laboratory uses the direct preparation then this result would be available in less than one week. The time to process the results therefore varies with the technique used by the laboratory; but specimens also take differing lengths of times to grow. Laboratory work on the samples is time-consuming, one technician processing only about five a week. Overload on laboratory resources often delays the results. Generally, the result is available by 13 weeks of pregnancy, which is still up to seven weeks earlier than amniocentesis.

TEST FAILURE

If CVS is unsuccessful it is for one of two reasons — the operator failed to obtain an adequate specimen (technical failure) or the laboratory failed to produce an adequate result (laboratory failure).

Both of these failure rates are higher with CVS than with amniocentesis. Only about 1 per cent of women who have an amniocentesis will need a repeat test, whereas with CVS it is between 2 and 10 per cent, being closer to 2 per cent in expert hands.

CVS can be a more difficult technique than amniocentesis, hence the higher technical failure rate. With experience, the operator learns to circumvent the difficulties or anticipate difficulties that are likely to result in a failed test. Even so, experienced centres have a failure rate of between 1 per cent and 6 per cent for transcervical CVS and about 1.5 per cent for transabdominal CVS.

Difficulties are expected with a transcervical approach if there is a sharp bend in the cavity of the uterus or cervix. In early pregnancy the axis of a pregnant woman's uterus can be sharply bent forwards (anteverted) or backwards (retroverted). A fibroid (a thickening of the wall of the uterus) may cause a similar obstruction if it is low in the uterus, rendering the test difficult or impossible. The most difficult transabdominal CVS is the unusual situation in which the uterus is tilted backwards (retroverted) and all of the placenta inserted into the back wall of the uterus. With experience, most of the difficulties discussed above may be circumvented.

Occasionally the laboratory receives a good specimen but none of the cells from the placenta grow. This happens in up to 2 per cent of specimens and prevents chromosome analysis. If the test does fail, the alternatives are to repeat the CVS or have an amniocentesis. Whichever of the two methods is chosen, seldom does the second specimen fail to grow.

There are an additional two potential sources of error which can cause confusing results. Maternal cell contamination is when cells from the pregnant woman, rather than from the fetus, grow. Now that laboratories have become experienced at processing samples and meticulously removing any of the pregnant woman's tissues from the specimen, this is a rare occurrence. Another occasional problem is mosaicism. This is when different cells analysed in the laboratory have differing chromosomes, a condition occurring in a small percentage of people. The outcome for the fetus depends on what the chromosome types are and the proportion of each type of cell. The CVS may occasionally show mosaicism even when it is not present in the fetus. Experts often have a good idea whether the mosaicism is likely to be affecting the fetus by looking at the pattern of the mixture of cells. Some mixtures of cells seen after CVS are so rare in live-born babies that further testing usually shows that it is not present.

Mosaicism occurs in approximately 1 per cent of CVS tests and can readily be sorted out if an amniocentesis is performed.

Occasionally the test results are ambiguous or later prove to be incorrect. These may be 'false positives', when an abnormal result is obtained in a normal fetus, or 'false negatives', when a normal result is obtained in a fetus with abnormal chromosomes. Most false positives are quickly detected by the laboratory as the abnormality is not seen in living pregnancies and follow-up amniocentesis is recommended. False negatives are very rare indeed.

Table 7.2 summarizes the chance of failure of CVS attributable to the causes outlined above. It shows that 2.2–10 per cent of women will require further testing either with a repeat CVS or amniocentesis. The chance that further testing is required depends mostly on the expertise of the doctor, as technical failures are potentially the largest group — it is at the lower end of the range in most experienced centres.

TABLE 7.2 REASONS FOR FAILURE OF CVS TESTING

Inadequate or no specimen	1–6%
Cells do not grow	0.4–2%
Doubtful result	0.8–2%
Total	2.2–10%

CVS IN MULTIPLE PREGNANCY

CVS can be performed in twin pregnancies, but not usually if there are three or more fetuses. It is reasonable to perform CVS on twins if there are clearly two placentas, both of which are accessible. In general, however, many believe twins to be a relative contraindication to the test.

Questions

Does CVS cause the fetus to move?

During CVS you may see the fetus moving on the ultrasound screen, but these movements are spontaneous — CVS has no influence on them. The needle is outside the pregnancy sac, so the fetus does not have any sensation or awareness of its presence.

Is CVS as accurate as amniocentesis?

If an abnormal result is produced with either test, it can be relied upon to be accurate. The doubtful CVS results are usually obvious to the laboratory, and they can nearly always be cleared up by having an amniocentesis later.

Can CVS detect as much as amniocentesis?

These two tests are as good as each other for diagnosing chromosomal abnormalities. Spina bifida cannot be diagnosed by CVS, but most people having a CVS are at very low risk of having a baby with spina bifida. Spina bifida can also be diagnosed with ultrasound.

Do more people choose CVS or amniocentesis?

The most popular choice depends on local expertise. In centres with expertise in CVS it is found that more and more women are choosing this method.

Can my cells grow at CVS, instead of those of the fetus?

While this can happen, with modern techniques it very rarely does.

Can I have CVS if I have been bleeding?

A woman who has vaginal bleeding in early pregnancy has an increased chance of miscarriage, even when the pregnancy appears healthy on ultrasound. Her 'background' risk is therefore higher than that of a woman who has had no bleeding. Whether performing a CVS in this situation also results in an increased risk of the test itself is uncertain. One reasonable policy is that if there has been no bleeding in the week prior to the proposed CVS, and the pregnancy appears healthy on ultrasound, then the test is unlikely to cause an increased risk of miscarriage.

If miscarriage occurs after CVS when would it happen?

Because miscarriages occur whether or not you have a CVS, there is no clear answer to this question. A miscarriage can occur at any time and there is no way of telling if the CVS caused it. Overall, there is a slight increase in the miscarriage rate after either CVS or amniocentesis. It is usually recommended that you reduce your level of activity for the 12 to 24 hours following CVS, but after this time there is little purpose in taking extra precautions.

Which is safest — transcervical or transabdominal CVS?

There is little difference in the risks of these two techniques. The risks depend more on the level of experience and skill of the person performing the procedure. The doctor who is to carry out your test could tell you his or her results.

No-Risk Tests for Down Syndrome

The tests for Down syndrome discussed in this chapter involve no risk to the fetus but are less accurate than CVS and amniocentesis. They are 'screening tests', and if the results are positive, further testing with either CVS or amniocentesis will be required to confirm whether any abnormality is present. The no-risk tests are able to detect only some of those fetuses with Down syndrome, but they have become increasingly popular.

It would be wonderful if Down syndrome could be diagnosed by a simple test, such as an analysis of the blood of the pregnant woman. We are a long way from this ideal, but some non-invasive tests that can indicate whether there is an increased risk of Down syndrome are now available. In this chapter we will look at what is currently possible and what might be possible in the future.

Amniocentesis and CVS are now widely available, low-risk tests for accurate diagnosis of chromosomal abnormalities. If you are at increased risk of carrying a fetus with a chromosomal abnormality, these techniques are available to you. If, however, like 90 per cent of the population, your chance of carrying an affected fetus is very small, the range of 'no-risk' tests may appeal to you more.

It seems contradictory, given that a woman's risk of carrying a Down syndrome fetus increases with her age, that most Down syndrome babies are born to young women considered to be at low risk. This is because women usually have their children before the age of 35, when their individual risk level is low. Together, these younger pregnant women give birth to 65 per cent of Down syndrome babies. If the prenatal detection rate of Down syndrome is to be improved, all pregnant women must be offered some other screening test.

A test that involved simply analysing the blood of the pregnant woman would be ideal; especially if it was cheap enough to allow all pregnant women to have it performed. Such screening tests are not perfect. They miss some Down syndrome fetuses and give some 'false positive' results, that is, an abnormal result when the fetus is actually normal. Women with an 'abnormal' blood test are offered amniocentesis or CVS to confirm the diagnosis. The aim is to improve the detection rate for fetuses with chromosomal abnormalities, not to detect all those affected.

Two types of blood tests have been suggested as screening methods for Down syndrome. The first involves looking for cells from the placenta and fetus that escape into the pregnant woman's circulation. The second, known as serum screening, is based on analysis of proteins and hormones that cross from the fetus into the pregnant woman's circulation.

Other non-invasive screening tests for Down syndrome include ultrasound scanning and one that is being researched — 'washings' from the cervix of the pregnant woman.

BLOOD TESTS

Fetal Cells in the Pregnant Woman's Circulation

Throughout pregnancy cells from both the placenta and the fetal blood enter the pregnant woman's circulation. These cells pass into the veins around the uterus and travel up towards the woman's heart. They are then pumped with the blood through the lungs and to the rest of the body. Using DNA techniques, chromosome abnormalities in the fetus have been detected from an analysis of fetal cells in the pregnant woman's blood. At present effective methods of concentrating the cells from the fetus have not been developed, and this is limiting the advancement of the technique. It is likely that these blood-screening methods will become more useful in time, although abnormal results may still need to be confirmed with amniocentesis or CVS.

Serum-screening Tests

Down Syndrome

It has been shown that a combination of blood tests on pregnant women, taken at 15 to 18 weeks, provides a cost-effective method of screening for Down syndrome. It is known that the blood of a woman carrying a Down syndrome fetus tends to contain slightly different levels of some substances, including alpha fetoprotein (AFP); human chorionic gonadotrophin (HCG) — the hormone that is measured in a pregnancy test; and an oestrogen called 'unconjugated oestriol'. A combination of the age of the pregnant woman, high levels of HCG, and low levels of AFP and unconjugated oestriol has to date provided the best method of screening all pregnant women for Down syndrome.

The test is usually called 'positive' if the risk of Down syndrome is one in 250 or more (this is a risk ratio equivalent to that of a 37-year-old woman). Approximately 5 per cent of pregnant women are offered amniocentesis as a result of a 'positive' test, and 60 per cent of Down syndrome fetuses are detected using this method. About 1 in 50 of those women with a positive result who are offered amniocentesis will be shown to be carrying a Down syndrome fetus. Clearly, most pregnant women with abnormal serum-screening results are found to be carrying a normal fetus, but the chance of Down syndrome being present is increased.

Attention is currently focused on developing a blood test for the pregnant woman that can be carried out much earlier, such as in the third month. These are only starting to become available, and are not yet as accurate as testing at 15 to 18 weeks.

Neural Tube Defects

Alpha-fetoprotein (AFP) is a protein made by the fetus that circulates in its bloodstream to help maintain fluid balance. Tiny amounts of AFP cross into the pregnant woman's circulation during pregnancy, the levels rising in early pregnancy.

For many years the level of AFP in the amniotic fluid has been used as an indicator for neural tube defects — spina bifida and anencephaly. In spina bifida there is an opening in the skin between the spinal canal and the amniotic fluid, and in anencephaly the skull bones do not form. The level of AFP is very much higher in the cerebrospinal fluid (the fluid around the spinal cord and brain), so a neural tube defect causes more AFP to pass into the amniotic fluid. This results in a higher amount finding its way into the pregnant woman's circulation.

Many countries routinely offer maternal serum AFP tests (which analyse the level of alpha-fetoprotein in the pregnant woman's blood) at 15 to 18 weeks. This allows the detection of 95 per cent of fetuses with anencephaly and 70 per cent of those with spina bifida.

Even when this test indicates a high level of AFP in the woman's blood, the fetus usually does not have a neural tube defect. It functions as a screening test, and as such does not aim to be 100 per cent accurate, but simply to select those fetuses that require further testing. Occasionally other factors, such as a multiple pregnancy or a deficiency in the abdominal wall of the fetus (an exomphalos), may cause a raised maternal serum AFP. It may also indicate a pregnancy that is further advanced than expected.

If the maternal serum AFP is high, further tests are carried out, the first being an ultrasound examination. This will detect many of the causes, including spina bifida, anencephaly, twins, or an exomphalos. If the ultrasound gives a normal result, and the fetal size is appropriate for dates, then amniocentesis may be suggested to test the AFP in the amniotic fluid. Usually, however, ultrasound will identify any spina bifida.

Serum Screening Programs

The major problem with serum screening programs is the technical one. Pregnant women need to be advised of the program and its implications in advance, because not all pregnant women wish to have tests for spina bifida and Down syndrome. A good laboratory service is essential as these are very sensitive tests, and unless the laboratory is well organised and carrying out a large number of tests, it is difficult for it to define its normal ranges clearly enough for accurate testing. Results are also improved if an ultrasound examination is carried out before the blood test to assess accurately the age of the pregnancy.

Serum screening is a complex process, and it can be difficult for couples to understand the implications of a positive result. Most women expect to be reassured by the test, and the possibility of a positive result and the subsequent consequences are often not considered beforehand. It has been shown that women who receive a positive result experience a high level of anxiety, possibly even higher than that experienced by people about to undergo surgery. This is partly because people are used to the result of a medical test being either 'positive' or 'negative'; positive confirming that there is disease present, negative confirming that there is not. But serum screening is not so clear cut. Approximately 5 per cent of pregnant women will receive a positive result, but most of these do not carry a fetus with Down syndrome. Alternatively, some women with a negative result do carry a fetus with Down syndrome. However, the perception of most couples is that a positive test indicates a problem. Around 49 out of 50 women with a positive result will not have a fetus with Down syndrome. If the fetus does not have the condition, the test is described as a 'false positive'.

Pregnant women who receive a positive result have been shown to experience raised levels of anxiety even after an amniocentesis has shown that Down syndrome is not present. Women often indicate that this anxiety is based on the premise that 'where there is smoke, there is fire'. This logic is understandable, but incorrect. Serum screening is a test, and a crude one, which indicates when there is a risk of Down syndrome. If your test is positive, and the fetus is subsequently shown not to have the condition, there is no increased risk for the remainder of the pregnancy.

Another difficulty with the screening program, which perhaps also explains the high level of anxiety experienced by many couples, is that the tests are currently not performed until 15 to 18 weeks of pregnancy. By the time the results of the blood tests are available, plus those of a follow-up amniocentesis when indicated, the pregnancy is likely to have progressed to almost 20 weeks. Although an abortion is medically possible at any stage of pregnancy, a termination at this late stage is emotionally traumatic for the couple involved. This situation will be improved soon, when serum screening tests taken at around 10 weeks become available, but these are still being tested to determine their accuracy. Couples will then have the results before the end of the third month of pregnancy. With fewer delays in the system there will be much less stress and anxiety for couples awaiting the results.

A 'Positive' Serum Screening Test

A 'positive' test result may be due to a raised serum AFP that indicates an increased chance of the fetus having a neural tube defect. Alternatively, a 'positive' result may indicate that the chance of the fetus having Down syndrome is higher than one in 250.

What Could Cause a Positive Result?

Only occasionally does a positive serum screening test mean that the fetus has an abnormality, such as Down syndrome or spina bifida. The most common causes of a positive result are:

(i) The pregnancy is either more or less advanced than expected (the interpretation of the result depends on the precise number of weeks of pregnancy).

(ii) Normal variations in the level of the substances in the pregnant woman's blood.

What Further Tests are Available?

If you receive a positive serum screen result you will be offered further tests, including:

(i) Ultrasound examination: this shows the age of the pregnancy and whether there is more than one fetus. It also can detect some birth defects, including all cases of anencephaly and most instances of spina bifida. If the ultrasound shows that the age of the pregnancy is different from what was expected, the screening test may need to be reinterpreted and may no longer be regarded as positive.

(ii) Amniocentesis or CVS: each of these will test for Down syndrome; amniocentesis also tests for neural tube defects (see chapters 6 and 7).

If There is an Abnormality will It be Detected?

If there is a chromosome abnormality, it will virtually always be detected by amniocentesis or CVS. Ultrasound can detect spina bifida in over 95 per cent of cases, so although this abnormality can also be diagnosed using amniocentesis, most couples whose fetus is at increased risk of spina bifida decide not to have amniocentesis if the spine appears normal on the scan.

What If an Abnormality is Present?

If further testing confirms the presence of an abnormality, the results will be discussed with you and your partner, and information will be provided about the type of abnormality present and how it might affect the baby after birth. The option of termination of pregnancy will also be discussed.

It is important to remember that although a positive serum screening test indicates a higher than average risk of Down syndrome or spina bifida, most women with positive tests go on to have a normal, healthy baby.

CERVICAL WASHINGS

Placental (or trophoblast) cells can be obtained by passing a fine catheter into the cervix of the pregnant woman, injecting a small amount of fluid, and then drawing the fluid up into the syringe. The cells obtained include some from the placenta and some from around the cervix and the lower part of the uterus. If a pure sample of these cells could be prepared, they could be cultured and analysed for Down syndrome and other chromosome abnormalities. The difficulty at the moment is to obtain a pure sample, so this test is still in the research stages.

ULTRASOUND TO DETECT DOWN SYNDROME
At 18 to 20 weeks

Some extravagant claims have been made about the accuracy of ultrasound detection of Down syndrome at 18 to 20 weeks. It has been suggested that by looking at a series of signs, such as fluid at the back of the neck, the length of the long bones, the amount of fluid in the kidneys, and the appearance of the bowel, 80 per cent of fetuses with Down syndrome can be detected. Another claim has been that by looking for subtle holes in the heart (ventricular septal defects), 90 per cent of fetuses with Down syndrome can be detected.

In reality, those who have reported large series of patients have shown that a smaller percentage of the fetuses with Down syndrome are detected at an 18–20-week scan. It is safest to assume that few Down syndrome fetuses would be detected at this stage — if an ultrasound centre detects 1 in 3 fetuses at 18 to 20 weeks it is doing well.

At 10 to 13 Weeks

One of the most important findings in recent times has been that at 10 to 13 weeks at least 60 per cent of fetuses with Down syndrome have a fluid layer of 3mm or more at the back of the neck, known as nuchal oedema. This is a transient finding — if these fetuses are scanned again at 18 weeks they will nearly always appear normal and the fluid layer will have resolved. A scan at 10 to 13 weeks is therefore increasingly being offered to pregnant women, especially those of 35 years and over who do not wish to have amniocentesis or CVS. If the chromosomes are normal and the fluid layer only a little thickened, the fetus is just a little slower to remove fluid from the head and neck area at this early stage of pregnancy and will appear normal at birth.

Women over 35 years of age who choose not to have an amniocentesis or CVS to test for Down syndrome may request an ultrasound at 10 to 13 weeks and expect at least 60 per cent of the Down syndrome fetuses to be detected. A scan at 10 to 13 weeks has been shown to be the best screening test for Down syndrome (that is, better than blood tests) for women of all ages, but only if measured carefully, using a standard method, and taking into account the number of weeks of pregnancy and the age of the pregnant woman. This level of expertise is not yet widely available. A combination of a scan at 10 to 13 weeks and early serum screening appears to be the way of the future for Down syndrome testing.

Questions

Surely there must be something wrong if the serum screening test is abnormal?

It is not correct to think of the test as looking for an abnormality, it is a screening test to indicate when there is a higher risk of an abnormality being present. More than 95 per cent of pregnant women who have a test outside the normal range have an absolutely healthy baby.

If there is an abnormality causing the high or low serum screening test, will it always be found?

If the serum screening test shows that the fetus has an increased risk of Down syndrome, the amniocentesis or CVS will confirm whether or not the condition is present. If the AFP level is high, ultrasound can be expected to detect around 95 per cent of those fetuses with spina bifida. If no neural tube defect is seen, some doctors would suggest an amniocentesis, which occasionally detects a spina bifida missed on the scan. It is most unlikely that a fetus with Down syndrome or spina bifida would be missed if appropriate follow-up testing with ultrasound and possibly amniocentesis is undertaken.

chapter 9

Ethics of Prenatal Testing

Many ethical issues surround the practice of prenatal test-ing. This book presents information, not moral arguments for and against the procedures, because we believe it is important for women and their partners to be aware of the issues and to discuss them with each other and their doctors. This chapter introduces some of the ethical and legal aspects of testing, abortion, the doctor's role, and counselling.

Prenatal testing gives women the opportunity to exclude some of the uncertainties and anxieties surrounding pregnancy. But it also raises questions that need to be discussed within society. Now that the technology is widely available and relatively safe, should every couple have the right to testing? What role should doctors play in giving advice in such a medically and ethically complex area? How should couples react when queries are raised by chromosome analysis, or when it is difficult to predict how a child will be affected by a diagnosed abnormality? We will look briefly at some of the ethical concerns of prenatal diagnosis and at the kind of counselling you should expect. For those interested in more information, a list of further reading is included at the end of this book.

SHOULD THE RIGHT TO TESTING BE UNIVERSAL?

By far the largest group of women having babies are those under 35 years of age who have no previous history of genetic abnormalities. For these women, the chance of carrying a fetus with a chromosome abnormality is so low that most do not wish to accept the additional, although slight, risk of miscarriage carried by genetic testing. Unless there are other indications, such as a previous baby with a chromosome abnormality, most women of this age are limited to testing with ultrasound and serum screening. There are some women below the age of 35, however, who are so anxious about the risk of abnormalities that they ask for further testing. The reasoning of Penny, who at 33 had an amniocentesis for her first child, illustrates the difficulty involved in imposing strict age limits.

> I had done a lot of work with children with intellectual disabilities and a number of their parents were quite young. Just because I was a couple of years younger than the usual testing time I didn't think that was sufficient insurance. I knew my life options would mean continuing working, and having a disabled child would make this difficult. I had thought through the issue, and I decided I was prepared to terminate the pregnancy if it was a Down syndrome fetus.

The results were normal, but unfortunately Penny's baby was still-born. Pregnant again a year later, she once more pushed for testing, despite the trauma of having already lost a baby.

> I knew it would be awful, but just because I had lost one baby didn't mean I wanted a disabled child. There was a lot of opposition from women in my support group who had also lost babies. Some were so desperate to have another child, they said: 'Give me one no matter what is wrong with it.' I still wasn't considered to be in the high-risk group and it was much harder to get a test than 12 months before. My obstetrician was supportive, but he had to sales-talk the pathologist and operator.

Situations such as Penny's have raised a major question for service providers: should there be a strict age limit for prenatal testing, or should couples be free to choose? Because of the labour-intensive and expensive nature of the laboratory processing, many centres have imposed fairly strict criteria on the availability of tests. Recently, however, there has been a tendency for greater flexibility, particularly with privately insured patients.

On the surface, it seems more equitable to give all couples who wish to undergo the procedures the right to do so. But there are arguments against making testing more readily available. It has been suggested that if women are offered such tests when in the emotionally vulnerable state of pregnancy, it may be difficult for them to make an informed decision based on the relative risks and benefits — this is known as the 'technological imperative'. Studies have shown, however, that most pregnant women at low risk do say no if offered testing, but offering the tests increases their autonomy.

Another argument is based on the cost of prenatal testing, which in most Western countries is roughly equivalent to an average week's wage. If the public health system bears the cost, governments expect to see a cost benefit from the testing, and this is difficult to demonstrate in low-risk groups.

IS ABORTION FOR ABNORMALITY ETHICAL?

Pregnancy termination is the option chosen by most Australian pregnant women who are found to be carrying a fetus with a major abnormality. Surveys taken in Australia indicate that this practice is widely supported. One study showed that 86 per cent of people believed that legal abortion was acceptable in cases where the fetus has an abnormality. This figure remained stable across the boundaries of age, sex and education level of those surveyed, with Protestants showing 90 per cent acceptance and Catholics 76 per cent. A similar acceptance rate applies in the UK (85 per cent) and USA (75 per cent).

Ethicists, like other members of the general public, differ in their views about abortion. The Roman Catholic Church believes that at any stage of pregnancy, from the moment of conception, abortion is a form of homicide. However, this view only became widely held from the nineteenth century. Earlier Christian philosophers said the soul entered the fetus at 'quickening', which was believed to be 40 days after conception for males and 80 days for females.

Some ethicists believe that when the fetus is able to survive independently from the pregnant woman it should have the same right to life as a child. With currently available paediatric intensive care facilities this occurs at approximately 24 weeks. While many medical practitioners, and indeed many members of the general public, see 20 weeks as the upper limit at which pregnancy termination may be legally and ethically performed, this milestone appears to have little ethical or legal basis.

Finally, there are ethicists who advocate that the fetus does not have a right to life until as late as 28 days after birth. This is based on the philosophy that before this time the infant could not possibly have a sense of its own existence and that this sense is a precondition to a right to life.

A consensus between the divergent views on the ethics of abortion is unlikely to be reached. Therefore, a decision on whether abortion is acceptable when a fetus has been diagnosed with an abnormality, or indeed in any other situation, remains a complex and personal one.

IS ABORTION FOR ABNORMALITY LEGAL?

Abortion laws vary around Australia. In Victoria and New South Wales, where there is no legal limit on when an abortion may be performed, the common law ruling indicates that abortion is lawful if performed solely to preserve the life and good health of the pregnant woman. Fetal abnormality itself is not specifically a ground for termination of pregnancy. However, the anticipation of delivering a baby with a major abnormality undoubtedly causes great emotional and psychological stress in the pregnant woman. It is this fact, rather than the abnormality itself, that forms the legal basis for the pregnancy termination.

South Australia and the Northern Territory have legislation making it lawful to perform pregnancy termination where there is a substantial risk that the child would be seriously disabled. In this case, the presence of the abnormality itself makes the termination legal.

WHICH FETUS CAN BE TERMINATED?

We have seen that both the community and the law support the termination of pregnancies in which the fetus has a severe abnormality. As the resolution of ultrasound equipment becomes more sophisticated, increasingly minor abnormalities are being detected. We have now reached the stage where we can detect a cleft (or 'hare') lip, which is readily treatable, usually with an excellent cosmetic result. Other relatively minor abnormalities that can be detected include misshapen (or 'club') feet and missing fingers. Since in Victoria and New South Wales abortion cannot legally be performed for the abnormality itself, but rather because the abnormality is deemed to risk the psychological health of the pregnant woman, then an abortion for such minor abnormalities may be said to be legal. Many practitioners would be prepared to follow the wishes of the pregnant woman and terminate the pregnancy if asked to do so, even though some would argue that the pregnant woman is making an irrational decision. If the doctor's own moral views prevent him or her from participating in a termination for a minor abnormality, the pregnant woman could be referred to a doctor prepared to carry out the abortion.

Sex selection is undoubtedly one of the most controversial areas of prenatal diagnosis. Many practitioners fear that couples may use knowledge of the sex of the fetus as a basis for termination of the pregnancy if the sex was not in accordance with their wishes. In a survey of medical geneticists in 18 nations it was found that only 25 per cent would be prepared to perform an abortion on the grounds of sex selection, and this was seen as their area of greatest ethical conflict. Many of those prepared to carry out sex selection argued that they would agree to it on the basis that without sex selection such women would terminate the pregnancy anyway.

Pregnancy termination on the grounds of sex is very rare in Australia. In almost two decades of prenatal diagnosis practice, only an extremely small number of patients have requested or enquired about sex selection. Most have been enquiries only and have not progressed to actual requests. Typical was a woman who already had five sons and arrived with a letter from a psychiatrist indicating that her psychiatric health would be at risk if sex selection was not permitted. However, like many such enquiries, an actual request for testing did not ensue.

WHAT ROLE SHOULD DOCTORS PLAY?

Two of the major dilemmas facing doctors working in prenatal diagnosis are being able to strike a balance between full disclosure of information and causing inappropriate anxiety, and the issue of nondirective counselling. Everybody agrees in principle with the full disclosure of results to pregnant women. But there are borderline situations, such as a mosaic result at CVS indicating the presence of only one or two abnormal cells as against 150 normal ones, which are extremely unlikely to have any impact on the baby. However, even though a doctor will try to explain this, couples commonly have such a fear of abnormality that they see the slightest suggestion of a problem as confirming their worst fears. Medically, the result may be of no significance, but conveying this to parents can be difficult.

A case that illustrates this point is the distress experienced by Margaret, whose fetus was found at amniocentesis to have a pericentric inversion of chromosome 9. She was assured that this inversion was considered a normal variant and had never been known to produce any abnormalities in babies. Family members were tested for the inversion, and the variant was found in both her husband and his mother. This did not reassure Margaret — in fact, she began looking for signs in their personalities and physical attributes that might be associated with the inversion. At one stage, she wondered whether it might be connected with the fact that both had some hearing problems. She worried throughout the pregnancy, until the baby was born and seen to be normal and healthy.

Most doctors involved in prenatal diagnosis strongly advocate non-directive counselling; that is, that results, risks and options should be presented as objectively as possible. Even with the best will in the world, it is often difficult for a counsellor to avoid indicating his or her views. Many of the concepts involved are complex and couples tend to seek direction from experts in the field.

Patients or Customers?

The debate about whether people who visit doctors are patients or customers highlights the developing consumerism in medicine. There is a new focus on caring for the needs of individuals and an expectation that patients will ask penetrating questions about the services they are receiving. Many of us welcome this change.

The prime concern of those practising ultrasound has often been with the technology. The pace of technological development in diagnostic ultrasound has been extremely swift. Such advances have allowed practitioners to glean increasing amounts of information on the normal and abnormal anatomy, and the physiological function, of the human body. However, ultrasound practice can become devoid of human warmth. As practitioners focus on technology and pathology, consideration of the whole person can be overlooked. Technology provides doctors with an extraordinary ability to assess the disease but not to care for the person.

It is time to consider how pregnant women respond to the diagnostic services provided to them, and to examine the difference that these services make to the overall well-being of the woman. Examples of unacceptable practices in prenatal diagnosis include women being unable to see the TV monitor during their ultrasound examinations and doctors not telling women immediately of any abnormal results. The obligation to provide a competent service does not preclude offering that service in a caring environment.

WHAT COUNSELLING SHOULD YOU EXPECT?

The information pregnant women receive is likely to influence their decisions for life. No book can replace discussions with your doctor or with the practitioner carrying out the tests. With invasive testing, such as amniocentesis and CVS, you should have the opportunity to discuss any aspects that concern you in advance. Rather than waiting until the day of the test, try to make an appointment for discussion beforehand so that you have time to consider all of the information. On the day of the test most people feel too anxious to focus on the important issues. It is standard in the USA and in some parts of Australia to have a separate interview with the practitioner before the tests are carried out. If this is not offered in the centre you will be attending, you may request it. Invasive tests carry a risk, and it is important that you fully understand the risks and benefits involved beforehand.

Many couples find it difficult to take the responsibility for making decisions about prenatal tests. Counselling provides an opportunity for couples to discuss their fears and anxieties, work through the issues, and come to an informed decision. Once couple illustrates this point well. Jane, 36, and Richard came for a 10-week scan, and Jane was found to be carrying twins. They asked for counselling on the risks of any testing and on the options for termination if an abnormality was detected. Jane became distressed when she described the outcome of her previous pregnancy. The fetus had died some time between the amniocentesis and an ultrasound scan at 18 weeks. The couple felt that the amniocentesis had caused the death. Richard said he could not bear to see Jane go through the experience again and believed that she should not have another test. The couple went away to think about their options and returned three days later saying they could not sleep, they could not make the decision, and that someone would have to make it for them. The counsellor began by asking them if they had decided to have a test. The answer was yes. He then moved on to the risks of each test. They opted for amniocentesis as it carries the lowest risk, but they were frightened of the procedure and needed reassurance that they were unlikely to have another fetal death following it. By spending time with a counsellor, and being able to work through the issues involved, Jane and Richard were able to make their own informed decision.

WHAT IF THE RESULTS ARE BAD?

Extensive support services are needed when a couple is told that a fetal abnormality has been detected. The information usually comes when the pregnancy has progressed to between 12 and 20 weeks and the couple has already planned in detail for the arrival of their baby. The bad news is everyone's worst nightmare, and the initial reaction is shock and overwhelming distress. The pregnant woman and her partner become numbed and are often unable to absorb the information they are being given. At this first discussion, it is too early to fill in all the details, but it is important that the couple leaves with some perspective on the suspected condition. Is the 'abnormality' merely the result of a screening test that indicates that further investigation should be considered? Or is it a confirmed abnormality? How severe is it and how will it affect the baby?

The amount of information provided at the time of the ultrasound examination varies. If the abnormality has been detected by an obstetrician specialising in ultrasound, you are likely to be informed at once about the extent of the abnormality. If the diagnosis has been made in a radiology practice, the radiologist may not explain the abnormality, because this is considered to be the responsibility of your obstetrician. Whoever conducts the initial interview, the details of the findings will need to be reinforced by your obstetrician at a later date. The temptation to make an instant decision on pregnancy termination should be avoided. A full understanding of how the abnormality would affect the baby often requires discussions with experts in the relevant area, such as a cardiologist if it is a heart abnormality or a paediatric surgeon if it is an abdominal problem. It is important to have an ongoing relationship with your doctor or genetic counsellor at this difficult time so that the information you are receiving can be coordinated and discussed.

Pregnancy Termination

The choice of whether to terminate a pregnancy that involves a major abnormality is a very personal one. Once you feel that you have received as much information as possible on the extent of the abnormality, you will need to make your decision. What you decide to do will depend upon what you know about the severity of the abnormality, your own views about abortion, and your personal and family situation.

If you decide not to continue with the pregnancy, there are two ways in which the termination can be carried out. First, labour can be induced by the use of drugs such as prostaglandin, and delivery usually occurs within 24 hours. This method is lengthy, and is associated with varying degrees of pain, although pain relief is available if required. Second, the cervix can be dilated, either surgically or initially with drugs and then surgically, and the fetus and placenta removed from the uterus. This method is called dilatation and evacuation (D & E) and is carried out under anaesthetic. The choice of method depends upon the nature of the abnormality, available expertise, and your own preference.

Following the termination of pregnancy you will need ongoing support and further information. Do not hesitate to make an appointment to see your own doctor or genetic counsellor after the procedure. When the results of any tests carried out on the fetus become available, your doctor will be able to assess the implications of the abnormality and the likelihood of it recurring in future pregnancies. There are some excellent support groups available for couples who have had a pregnancy termination due to a fetal abnormality. Such groups can provide much-needed emotional and practical support to you at a time when you will be feeling vulnerable. Your doctor should be able to give you information on the groups operating in your area.

Making the Decisions

Your decisions about prenatal diagnosis must be made on personal grounds, they cannot be made by doctors. This chapter provides a step-by-step account of the risks and benefits associated with the range of options available. It examines the important role of your attitudes and beliefs in decision-making, and relates the experiences of some couples who have already travelled down the same path. Guidelines are provided to help you select the best and most appropriate medical care.

Prenatal testing differs from most other medical diagnosis. If you had woken up this morning with severe abdominal pain, you would have visited your doctor, been examined, and probably have undergone some tests. If a diagnosis of appendicitis was made you would have an operation on your doctor's recommendation. Since you had chosen a doctor you trusted, you would have readily undergone the tests and surgery. In this instance, the recommended treatment is based on the beliefs of your doctor as to the likely cause of your pain. Because many people have been treated with this problem before you, the doctor can confidently make clear recommendations to you. It might be argued that the doctor's approach is paternalistic, since you have not been offered treatment options, but as you have been diagnosed with an obvious case of appendicitis this is deemed to be the rational approach.

Prenatal diagnostic tests for fetal abnormality, however, require a different approach. You are pregnant and have no symptoms of disease. Should you let nature take its course and accept whatever child is delivered? Or should you put your already-loved and nurtured unborn baby at additional risk to exclude the existence of some abnormalities? If the tests detect an abnormality, there is usually no treatment. The only options open to you are to continue the pregnancy, knowing that the baby will be born with an abnormality, or to terminate the pregnancy. If you are firmly opposed to abortion and would under no circumstances request one, then there are few bene-fits involved in testing for abnormality, given the increased risk of miscarriage involved.

No third party, medical practitioner or not, can decide whether you should risk miscarriage in order to undergo diagnostic testing, nor can they decide the future of your pregnancy if an abnormality is detected. These decisions should be made on personal grounds, including your religious and moral beliefs and the desires and expec-tations of you and your family. In prenatal testing the prevailing ethic is the autonomy of the couple involved — that is, couples should be encouraged to make their own decisions based on the available infor-mation. However, it takes time and effort to understand the issues involved. It perhaps seems much easier to ask your doctor, who certainly understands the medical aspects, what he or she would recommend. Most doctors would be prepared to advise in this situa-tion, but in reality they are able to provide you with very little guidance — their religious, moral and family backgrounds, and their emotional investment in the pregnancy, differ from your own. You can accept the recommendation of your doctor, who is in a poor position to make decisions on your behalf, or you can research the issues yourself. This chapter aims to help you go through the decision-making process, and relates the experiences of some couples who have already considered their options.

SHOULD I HAVE A TEST?

There are two types of prenatal tests for chromosome abnormality: those that carry no risk to the pregnancy — ultrasound scans and blood tests; and those that carry some risk — CVS and amnio-centesis. Women of all ages are offered an ultrasound examination at 18 to 20 weeks, primarily as a test for fetal abnormality and to check dates. When performed by an expert, an additional ultrasound scan at 10 to 13 weeks is also a good test for Down syndrome, and at this time many other abnormalities may also be detected. Maternal serum screening is also an established test for Down syndrome.

At present more than 90 per cent of women who elect to have an invasive test are over 35, although this percentage is reducing as the uptake of serum screening and 10–13-week ultrasound examinations is increasing. The major condition that increases in frequency with age is chromosomal abnormality. Because Down syndrome is the most common chromosome abnormality, and a major cause of intellectual disability, discussions usually focus on this condition. For a pregnant woman at the age of 36, the probability of detecting Down syndrome is about one in 200, the same as the risk of miscarriage attributed to amniocentesis.Although many would consider that a simple comparison of these numbers is irrelevant, because having a miscarriage cannot be equated with delivering a baby with Down syndrome, historically this comparison has been used to justify offering amniocentesis and CVS only to women of 35 to 37 years and older. These procedures diagnose virtually all cases of chromosome abnormality. Alternatively, you may opt for one of the two no-risk tests that detect most, but not all, Down syndrome cases — serum screening and ultrasound at 10 to 13 weeks. Many fetuses with Down syndrome and other chromosome abnormalities have a subtle fluid swelling at the back of the neck at around 10 to 13 weeks. In at least six out of ten fetuses with Down syndrome this fluid layer is 3mm or more at 10 to 13 weeks, and can be detected by an ultrasound scan. If swelling is detected at this stage, a CVS is then offered. Most of the studies of this finding have been of women of 35 years and above, but if carefully measured and used with established charts in conjunction with the age of the pregnancy and of the woman, the test should also be accurate for younger women. Ultrasound at 18 to 20 weeks is less likely than an earlier scan to detect fetuses with Down syndrome.

Table 10.1 outlines the major factors you should consider in deciding whether an invasive test is right for you. Besides age, factors that will influence your decision include your attitudes towards the risks of the tests, abortion, and bringing up a child with abnormalities. Any previous experience with pregnancy loss or long-standing infertility will also have an enormous influence. Any history of genetic disorders in your family will also have an impact on your decision, even if there is no increased risk of the disorder occurring.

Assessment of Risks

The comparison of statistical risks is fraught with problems. While it is convenient to say that for a woman of around 36 of age the risk of miscarriage from amniocentesis is equal to that of detecting a Down syndrome fetus, in many ways this is a false comparison. Are the outcomes equal? On the one hand, there is the loss of a pregnancy, and on the other a lifetime spent looking after your disabled child. Studies have shown that many women are prepared to accept an even

TABLE 10.1 FACTORS TO CONSIDER BEFORE DECIDING WHETHER TO HAVE A TEST

	Amniocenteis/CVS	No test
Age <35*	Performed if the couple is especially concerned	Favoured by balance of risks
Age 35–36	Balance of risks depends on how the figures are assessed	
Age >37	Favoured by balance of risks	If refused for reasons below
Parents' attitude	Wish to lower the chance of raising a child with an abnormality, so would accept abortion *or* Wishes time to accept an abnormality if present	Would accept a baby no matter what *or* Absolute moral, religious or other objection to abortion *or* Objection to prenatal testing because it focuses on the disability not the baby's individuality
Risk of miscarriage	Accepts the low risk of test	Accepts no increased risk

* The age is usually taken as the age you will be at the time you are due to deliver.

higher risk of miscarriage to guard against bringing a baby with abnormalities into the world. For others, especially those who have spent years trying to conceive, had repeated miscarriages, or suffered the death of a baby, any additional risk may seem too high. If you belong to the latter group, you might consider relying on ultrasound carried out by an operator skilled at detecting the subtle signs of Down syndrome, plus maternal serum screening. This course of action allows the detection of many of those fetuses with major abnormalities, without putting your pregnancy at risk.

Attitudes Towards Abortion

As stressed earlier, decisions about testing should be made by you and your partner, not by your doctor. They should be made after the risks, limitations,and benefits involved have been fully explained to you. Clearly, you and your partner's attitude towards pregnancy termination is crucial when considering which tests are appropriate for you, because chromosomal abnormalities, if found, cannot be cured. You may face a choice as to whether to continue with the pregnancy.

Many doctors argue that it is unnecessarily risky to carry out testing unless you are prepared to terminate the pregnancy following an unfavourable diagnosis. Others, however, make strong arguments in favour of testing high-risk couples, even when the detection of an abnormality would not lead to pregnancy termination. If fetal abnormalities are detected, they may be easier to come to terms with during pregnancy rather than at the emotionally charged time of birth. Also, testing may allow couples who choose to raise a child with abnormalities to have time for preparation. For Wendy, who found she was carrying a fetus with Down syndrome, the test result gave her the chance to adjust her goals and expectations.

I was advised that it was medically unsound to have a test unless you were prepared to act on the result. This was because of the risk of miscarriage. So my decision to have an amniocentesis was not made lightly. When I eventually decided against termination, I found the testing had been very valuable. Through that knowledge I had the chance to reset my goals before Sarah was born. In my decision-making, I had the normal dream of a child who would go to university and have a successful, happy life. Many parents' hopes are dashed anyway on those dreams. Instead of that, I had the time to develop positive alternatives to build on. At least, she wouldn't have a mortgage or any broken marriages.

Being aware that an abnormality exists may also help medical management in the following ways:

(i) Treatment can be carried out prior to birth for some conditions, such as urinary blockage and rapid heart rate.

(ii) Couples have the opportunity to prepare psychologically for the birth of a baby with a problem, including the opportunity to seek information from an appropriate expert (for example, a paediatric surgeon if a harelip has been diagnosed).

(iii) Allow delivery to be organized at the optimal time and in the appropriate manner (for example, it is safest for babies with some abnormalities to be delivered by caesarean section).

(iv) Arrange for the birth to take place at a specialist centre so that experts and specialist equipment are available if immediate treatment is needed.

It will help if you and your partner discuss beforehand what course you would take in the case of an abnormal result. As mentioned earlier, even if you are opposed to abortion, testing can be helpful. The odds favour a normal result, which will help reduce some of your anxieties, but if the result is abnormal, you will have a valuable few months for preparation.

History of Genetic Disorders

For those couples who have previously had a child born with an abnormality, or who have a history of genetic disorder in their family, the decision to have testing is generally taken much more easily. In fact, many such couples would remain childless if it were not for the availability of prenatal testing. For couples who have previously had a baby with Down syndrome, the chance of a second baby with a chromosome abnormality rises to 1 per cent if the pregnant woman is under 30 years. Above this age, the risk is the normal one associated with the specific age. When she became pregnant at 30, Heather did not fall into any of the high-risk groups for testing. She gave birth to a baby with Trisomy 18 who died 23 hours later. Again pregnant at 33, she was immediately offered an amniocentesis.

> I definitely wanted one. Although my chances of having another baby with a chromosome abnormality had not increased, I was quite prepared to accept a miscarriage rate of one in 200 to avoid going through that awful time after the birth again. I think amniocentesis is a valuable test. I would have spent the whole pregnancy being worried if it were not for the reassurance of the test.

For women who have delivered a baby with one of a number of other abnormalities, the risk of recurrence is even higher: for spina bifida, it is 3 per cent after the first affected baby, unless folic acid is taken before and in early pregnancy. One woman, whose first two pregnancies resulted in the detection of spina bifida, terminated both. After three years she became pregnant again, this time with a risk of 10 per cent of recurrence. Without amniocentesis, she would not have chanced the third pregnancy. Luckily, the results were normal, as was the resulting child.

Those with a family history of a gene disorder can be at even greater risk. Maria and Sergio, both carriers of the thalassaemia gene defect, had a chance of one in four of having a child with thalassaemia major. Maria described a family member's experience with the condition:

> My cousin has been through hell. He's very sickly and has to have repeated blood transfusions. They don't give him much chance of living beyond thirty-two. I wouldn't want to put a child through that. If we didn't have the option of testing, we would not have had a family. I had decided to terminate if the results were bad. We were very lucky, and never had to exercise this option. It gave us great peace of mind and allowed us to go ahead and have three healthy children.

The Limits of Testing

An important point, which has been emphasized throughout this book, is that the decision to have testing and act upon the result only lowers your chances of having an abnormal baby. A normal test result does not guarantee a normal, healthy baby. Some major abnormalities cannot be detected by any prenatal tests, including ultrasound, and there may be complications later in pregnancy or during the birth that cannot be predicted. Many women lose sight of this in the euphoria of normal results. When Maria's first pregnancy was tested for thalassaemia, the results were normal.

> I had a fetal blood test when I was first pregnant at 24. It was terrible waiting the six days for the results. But we were ecstatic. She was fine, everything was fine. Then I lost her when she was stillborn at seven months for some reason unrelated to the test. It was a terrible shock.

SHOULD I HAVE AN AMNIOCENTESIS OR CVS?

In deciding which test to have, there are advantages on either side which you should weigh up. Table 10.2 outlines the differences between the two. The major advantage of amniocentesis is that it is still a safer method of testing than CVS. It is for this reason that people who have spent a long time trying to conceive often choose amniocentesis. This technique also has a lower technical failure rate and is slightly less prone to producing uncertain results, so fewer women who have amniocentesis will require repeat testing. The only time amniocentesis is always used is in the uncommon situation when there is a higher than usual risk of a specific abnormality that cannot be diagnosed by CVS. Spina bifida is such an abnormality (although ultrasound is an accurate way of detecting spina bifida so usually amniocentesis is unnecessary).

The disadvantage of amniocentesis is that it is performed relatively late in pregnancy, and it is not until 17 to 20 weeks that the diagnosis is obtained. By this stage you will have begun to look pregnant and may be aware of movements. If the fetus is abnormal and you choose to have the pregnancy terminated, it is therefore more emotionally distressing. It is also medically more difficult to abort a pregnancy at 20 weeks than it is at an earlier stage. The fetus can be removed surgically, by dilatation of the cervix and removal of the fetus and placenta from the uterus. Alternatively, there are drugs which can reliably bring you into labour at this late stage, but this process usually takes up to 24 hours. As you would be aware that the fetus is abnormal and could not survive, this is a very difficult experience. The method used depends on the abnormality, available expertise, and your own preference. Few operators are experienced at dilation and evacuation, and because little information can be obtained about the abnormality at postmortem examination after this method, it is difficult to counsel couples in future pregnancies. Many women, when counselled about having an amniocentesis, are not told what a termination will involve.

> I had already had one baby die soon after birth because of an extra chromosome. When the results came back from amniocentesis, my decision would be to terminate if necessary. But I don't think I appreciated what this meant. At 20 weeks, you have an almost viable baby. It got to the point that if it had had the same chromosome abnormality I decided I would go through the pregnancy and let it die at birth.

TABLE 10.2   FACTORS TO CONSIDER IN CHOOSING CVS OR AMNIOCENTESIS

	CVS	Amniocentesis
Risk of miscarriage from test	Approx. 1%	Approx. 0.5%
Usual time to have test	10–12 weeks	15–17 weeks
When results received	11–14 weeks (before woman looks pregnant or feels movements)	17–20 weeks (after woman has felt movements)
Discomfort	Usually mild	Minimal
Usual type of abortion if sought	Vaginal (curette only)	Bring on labour (prostaglandins) or dilatation and evacuation
Test failure (see table 7.2)	2.2–10%	Approx. 1%
Previous baby with spina bifida	No	Yes
Obstetric factors		
— previous caesarean sections	Preferred	Late diagnosis a disadvantage
— weak cervix needing a suture	Result back before suture	Result back after suture
Major advantage	Avoids late abortion	Lowest risk

Because the results of CVS are available so much earlier, this has become a popular test. Certainly women who have been unfortunate enough to have an abortion at 20 weeks because of an abnormality tend to choose a CVS subsequently.

> Our pregnancy was settled, and I was fit and healthy. It never occurred to us that anything could be wrong. We decided to have an amniocentesis, anyway. When the obstetrician rang, we thought it was to change the appointment. We couldn't believe Ben had a sex chromosome abnormality. The obstetrician had said termination would be difficult, but I didn't realize just how terrible it would be or that it would involve twenty hours of labour. It was particularly awful because of the drugs and the way it was induced. If I had known, I would have chosen a CVS.

Those who have undergone CVS have a marked reduction in the level of anxiety and depression from the time they obtain their results. This occurs even though they are still at risk of miscarriage. From this time they are able to become attached to their unborn baby. By contrast, those who have amniocentesis remain anxious until they receive their results at 20 weeks. Feelings of attachment are suppressed for half the pregnancy.

WHO SHOULD PERFORM THE TEST?

As a consumer you should feel relaxed about asking your doctor or operator for information on the quality of the service you will receive. You wouldn't buy a refrigerator without enquiring about its quality and whether it is appropriate for your needs. Why should pre-natal diagnosis be any different? Pregnant women are sometimes nervous about asking, and often do not know which questions to ask. The problem is exacerbated by the fact that different ultrasound scans require different skill levels. Some are simple, such as checking to see if the fetus is presenting head first in labour. Others are more difficult, such as diagnostic scans for identifying heart abnormalities. Here is a guide to what you should expect in terms of equipment and operator skill and experience.

Ultrasound

If the examination is being performed to check for abnormalities at the 18–20-week scan, or if there has been a complication of pregnancy, you should evaluate the service in the following ways:

(i) Cost of equipment: good equipment currently costs between $150 000 and $350 000. A new model is released every three to four years, although older models may be upgraded.

(ii) Training: how long has the doctor or operator been in practice? How long was spent in training? Courses require training of up to two years, but one year would be considered satisfactory. Doctors who have been in practice for a number of years may have acquired extensive expertise on the job.

(iii) Experience: how many scans does the doctor perform each year? One thousand pregnancy scans per year is a good level of experience.

(iv) Expertise: how many cases of fetal heart abnormality has the operator detected? These are relatively common (around one in 300 fetuses), but are one of the most difficult abnormalities to detect.

Other Procedures

The loss rate following prenatal diagnostic procedures such as CVS, amniocentesis, and fetal blood sampling (FBS) is closely related to operator experience. The risk factors for the various procedures quoted in this book assume that they are carried out by skilled and experienced operators. There is no magical formula that allows you to assess 'adequate experience'. The figures given below suggest the minimum number of procedures that you should expect an experienced operator to have carried out:

Procedure	Training	Maintenance
Amniocentesis	100	50
CVS	100	50
FBS	30	30

'Training' refers to the period during which the operator is learning the procedure, usually under the supervision of an experienced practitioner. 'Maintenance' refers to the minimum number of procedures that should be performed per year in order to maintain expertise.

Amniocentesis is usually the first procedure undertaken by trainees, and it usually takes about 100 procedures before they are able to cope well with the technique. The number of times a second needle insertion is required (which should be about 1 per cent), and the number of times the operator causes blood staining of the amniotic fluid (also about 1 per cent), reduce with experience, and each is associated with an increased risk of miscarriage.

The suggested number of CVS procedures that should be carried out for minimum training ranges between 100 and 400. There is a continued reduction in the fetal loss rate, even after the operator has performed hundreds of procedures.

A large study carried out in the USA has shown that the fetal loss rate after FBS ranges between 1 and 6.8 per cent. It has been suggested that the complication rate is highest in the first 30 procedures performed by any given operator. Minimum FBS figures shown above assume that at least 100 amniocentesis or CVS procedures are also being performed by the operator in both the training and the maintenance phases.

SHOULD I FIND OUT THE SEX?

A chromosome analysis also indicates the sex of the fetus and this is written on the laboratory report. Your doctor can tell you the sex if you want to know. There is a range of attitudes on this subject. Some say that knowing the sex will take some of the excitement out of the birth and begin the process of sex stereotyping even earlier. Others believe in having all of the information available.

SHOULD I HAVE AN ABORTION?

The decision to have an abortion ultimately lies with the couple involved. If you are unfortunate enough to get an abnormal result on the tests, you will want to know how seriously this will affect your child. Unfortunately, chromosome analysis will not always give a clear picture of the severity of the abnormalities. Ultrasound will assist in assessing structural abnormalities, but will indicate nothing about mental development or organ function. Expert advice from genetic counsellors or paediatric specialists will fill in some of the gaps, while many self-help groups will willingly share with you the experiences of couples raising children with abnormalities.

If the abnormality is one of the trisomies, such as Down syndrome, or a serious congenital defect like spina bifida, almost every couple decides to have an abortion. Most, if given a choice, do not want to bring severely intellectually or physically disabled children into the world. Even these severe abnormalities, which cause a marked reduction in the quality of life, cause much heartbreak for some couples trying to come to a decision about the future of the pregnancy. One woman, who eventually decided to terminate her pregnancy following a diagnosis of Down syndrome, said:

> *There are enormous ethical issues at stake if we are to say people shouldn't live because they don't meet expectations. But these are abstract ideas. I couldn't stand to watch a child of mine being treated as the intellectually disabled are in our society.*

There are very few women, like Wendy mentioned earlier, who make a decision to continue a pregnancy when there is a major abnormality. Her experiences, and the kind of research she undertook, may help you in your decision. At 42, Wendy discovered through amniocentesis that her first baby had Down syndrome.

> *The results came back in two weeks. I went though a process of gathering information so that my decision would be an informed one. I visited schools and centres for those with Down syndrome. I went out with social workers. Personally I couldn't see any difference between a fetus at five months and one at nine months and I wasn't going to take a life without knowing the extent of the disabilities. The situation was closely monitored with ultrasound to see if there were any major heart abnormalities. It seemed that it was 90 per cent sure that the heart and digestive system were normal. It took me ten days to decide. Knowing that she would have a reasonable quality of life, I believed I didn't have the right to take it. Just because she didn't reach the norm, should she be culled? Her father left me as soon as I made the decision. He couldn't cope and I didn't see him again until Sarah was born. I had prepared myself that she would be healthy and it was an excellent birth. Knowing she was a Down syndrome baby did not detract from the experience. My goals by then were different and I had reset all my aspirations for her. Her father came to the birth and once he saw her, I couldn't get her out of his arms. She's now six months old, a delightful little girl that her father sees once a week. I'm very happy about my decision.*

There are other conditions, such as sex chromosome abnormalities, where the range of disability is wider still. Some children may be intellectually normal, others impaired. This uncertainty presents couples with a difficult decision; about half decide to terminate, while the rest proceed with the pregnancy. If a couple desperately want a child, and have had trouble conceiving, they may find the risk of lower intelligence and infertility bearable. If, on the other hand, this is an accidental pregnancy, and the couple have several other healthy children, they may decide to terminate the pregnancy. Couples with strong academic interests and high expectations might not be able to cope with the idea of an intellectually impaired child.

The laws on abortion vary, but in practice they are usually liberally interpreted. As prenatal diagnosis technology increases in sophistication, couples may wish to terminate pregnancies for even more minor abnormalities. Much of the opposition to prenatal testing focuses on this point, the desire for 'perfect' babies. Where should the line be drawn?

If you decide to have an abortion following the diagnosis of an abnormality, it is likely to be a traumatic experience, particularly when it is a much-wanted baby. Some couples ask for the diagnosis to be confirmed after the abortion to ensure that a mistake has not been made. A postmortem examination can often be carried out, which gives some women and their partners reassurance that they have made the right decision. Whether at 12 or 20 weeks, abortion involves a great loss. Many women find that the community does not appreciate the bonding they have with an unborn baby, and they receive comments such as 'Don't worry, you'll have another one'. You will need time to say goodbye to the baby and to gather support around yourself and your partner. There are some support groups, such as Support After Fetal Diagnosis of Abnormality (SAFDA), that may be able to offer you some useful help during this difficult time. As with any loss, you are likely to go through a grieving process and have increased anxiety with future pregnancies.

Other Tests and Treatments Occasionally Used

In this book we have concentrated on ultrasound, serum screening, CVS and amniocentesis as these are the most widely used tests for abnormalities or genetic disease. The aim of this chapter is to complete the picture by examining other methods of visualizing the fetus and other invasive tests currently used or likely to be used in the near future. We will conclude with a short segment on treatment before birth of fetuses with abnormalities.

OTHER WAYS OF LOOKING AT YOUR FETUS
X-Rays

X-rays are still occasionally used in pregnancy, although ultrasound has usurped many of its roles. In the non-medical community there remains a widespread concern that X-rays during pregnancy may cause abnormalities or cancer later in childhood. While at high doses both of these can happen, using modern X-ray equipment the dose of irradiation is very low. It is now believed that X-rays used for diagnosis will not cause these problems, so abortion should not be recommended solely on the basis of exposure to diagnostic radiation.

X-rays are used for three purposes in pregnancy:

(i) To check the fetus for structural abnormalities, to see which way it is lying or to diagnose multiple pregnancy. Ultrasound has now virtually totally replaced the use of X-rays in these areas.

(ii) To examine the size of the pregnant woman's pelvis. Occasionally it is important to know the size of the pelvis before labour if, for example, the fetus is in a breech position (buttocks down), or if the pregnant woman has had a Caesarean section in an earlier pregnancy. Ultrasound is not able to measure the pelvic size. When these X-rays are carried out, as much of the fetus as possible is shielded from the X-rays so that it receives the minimum dose.

(iii) To investigate other diseases in pregnancy. If the pregnant woman has an illness in pregnancy, such as kidney disease, this may require investigation with X-rays. Wherever possible, the fetus is shielded when the X-rays are taken.

The general principle is that X-rays are only used if their potential benefit is likely to far outweigh any risks.

Magnetic Resonance Imaging (MRI)

This is a new and exciting tool for medicine which is likely to be used more and more. It has the advantage of showing tissue function whereas ultrasound cannot. The patient is placed in a large magnet, the magnet turned on and the energy released by the body's molecules measured when it is turned off. This very expensive equipment provides beautiful high-resolution images and is increasingly used for diagnosis of diseases. Its use in obstetrics has been limited because of the cost and because the still images produced are less versatile and useful than ultrasound. As it does not involve irradiation, it is believed to be safe, although it is not recommended in the first three months of pregnancy. More work has to be done in this area before the technique can be used widely on the fetus.

OTHER TESTS ON AMNIOTIC FLUID
For Infection

While most infections during pregnancy are known to be unlikely to damage the fetus, there are several that may. German measles (rubella) was the first infection demonstrated to produce abnormalities in the fetus and this still occurs occasionally in pregnancy. Other potentially damaging infections are cytomegalovirus (CMV) and toxoplasmosis, both more common, but less hazardous, than rubella. Rubella causes a rash, and CMV and toxoplasmosis a prolonged flu-like illness. If a pregnant woman has an illness suggestive of one of these, or comes into contact with somebody with the disease, she can have a blood test. If the blood test is positive, amniocentesis or fetal blood sampling may be suggested to see whether the fetus has developed the infection.

Amniocentesis may also be used to look for infection if the membranes rupture early. If this occurs, infection is able to spread up into the uterus from the vagina.

Another viral infection that can cause problems in the fetus is parvovirus (or 'slap face' virus). This can result in breakdown of the red blood cells, which sometimes requires a fetal blood transfusion before birth. Fetal damage can also occur following chickenpox.

For Blood Group Incompatibility

If there is a blood group incompatibility between the pregnant woman and the fetus (the commonest and best known is Rhesus or Rh incompatibility), routine tests on the pregnant woman's blood will detect it. Amniocentesis or fetal blood sampling is often used to assess the severity of anaemia in the fetus resulting from the blood group incompatibility. While these are performed late in pregnancy, the techniques and most of the risks are similar to those discussed in chapter 6 and in this chapter respectively.

For Lung Maturity

Lung immaturity of very premature babies presents their most common barrier to survival. Normal babies and adults produce fluid called surfactant, which lines the air spaces to the lungs and prevents their collapse. Babies do not produce surfactant until about 34 weeks or sometimes even later. When an infant is likely to deliver early, amniocentesis may be performed to test for the presence of this surfactant in the amniotic fluid as a means of indicating whether the baby is likely to have severe lung disease after birth. If surfactant is not present, an injection of steroids (cortisone) into the pregnant woman will cross the placenta and help the fetus to produce it.

FETAL BLOOD SAMPLING (FBS)

Fetal blood sampling is an ultrasound-guided technique (shown in figure 11.1) in which a needle is passed through the skin and uterus of the pregnant women and into a blood vessel of the fetus, usually in the umbilical cord, to withdraw blood. When used for chromosome testing, its major advantage is that a result is available in less than one week. The test is often called percutaneous umbilical blood sampling (PUBS) or cordocentesis. The main reasons for having FBS are:

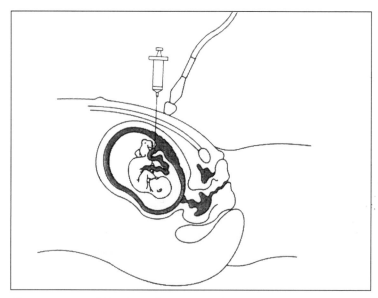

Figure 11.1   Fetal blood sampling: the needle is passed into a vessel in the cord, usually at a point 1–2 cm from the placenta.

(i)   an at-risk pregnancy (e.g. age greater than 35) where the woman presents too late to allow laboratory processing of chromosomes in an amniocentesis specimen;

(ii)   an abnormality found on ultrasound that may be the result of an underlying chromosomal abnormality;

(iii) a fetus at risk of a disease in which a blood test is required for diagnosis, e.g. some cases of haemophilia and thalassaemia;

(iv) some intrauterine infections, e.g. toxoplasmosis;

(v)   a fetus with markedly reduced growth, to test for an underlying chromosomal abnormality or for oxygen and carbon dioxide levels in the blood;

(vi) a major increase or decrease in amniotic fluid volume.

Timing of FBS

Fetal blood sampling may be performed at any time after 16 weeks. In general it becomes easier later in pregnancy. There has been a report of its use as early as 12 weeks, but the cord is very fine at this stage, and generally it is not carried out until later.

Who Should Perform the FBS?

A report in the *British Medical Journal* suggests that centres performing FBS should be doing at least 30 per year. Expertise is more easily maintained by a doctor whose practice includes amniocentesis and CVS. If you ask, the doctor should be able to give you an idea of the numbers performed and the miscarriage rate following the test in his or her practice.

The Procedure

A 20- to 22-gauge needle is passed under ultrasound guidance through the skin of the pregnant woman's abdomen, through the uterus and into the cord near the point where it connects with the placenta. The passage of the needle is either through the placenta and directly into the cord without entering the amniotic space, or into the amniotic space and then on into the cord. Once the needle is inside the cord it is manipulated until the tip enters one of the blood vessels and blood can be withdrawn into the syringe. Afterwards, the site in the cord that has been punctured is checked to ensure that bleeding is not occurring, and the fetal heartbeat is observed for any irregularity.

Blood may also be taken from a vessel within the body instead of the umbilical cord, or directly from the fetal heart.

From the pregnant woman's point of view this procedure differs little from amniocentesis. No special preparation is required before the fetal blood sample. The procedure may take longer than amniocentesis as the operator must place the tip of the needle into a vessel in the cord. Following FBS there is no need to stay in hospital but you will be advised to go home and rest.

Possible Complications

The most important complication of the test is death of the fetus due to the test. In experienced hands this occurs in approximately 1 to 2 per cent of cases. Other potential complications include persistent bleeding from the cord after withdrawal of the needle: bleeding usually stops within one minute. In rare cases there may be bleeding into the cord to produce a localized haematoma (blood collection). Following blood sampling the heart rate may slow, but it usually returns to normal soon after. Other potential complications are the same as for amniocentesis (see chapter 6).

BIOPSY OF THE FETUS

The precision provided by ultrasound allows a piece of tissue from the fetus to be removed with a needle. This is rarely done, but might be carried out, for example, to do a skin biopsy of a fetus that is at risk of a severe skin disease which would result in its death shortly after birth.

The procedure of skin biopsy is similar to amniocentesis, with ultrasound providing the means to place the tip of the biopsy forceps against the skin where a small piece is taken. With appropriate equipment this is not usually difficult and therefore is not an unduly risky procedure for the fetus, but because it is not commonly done, precise figures cannot be quoted. Usually little or no mark from where the skin was taken is visible after birth. Other parts may be biopsied, such as the liver, but this is rarely called for.

FETOSCOPY

Ultrasound-guided procedures have virtually replaced fetoscopy, the passage of a telescope-like instrument through the abdomen and into the uterus to allow direct visualization of the fetus, cord and placenta.

It has been used since 1973 for taking blood or other tissues, and for looking at some abnormalities which are difficult to diagnose using any other method. This procedure was technically difficult and took a great deal of experience, and the risk of miscarriage after the test was much higher than with ultrasound-guided procedures. Since the improved resolution of ultrasound equipment has allowed the detection of most abnormalities visualized by fetoscopy there is now little place for this technique.

EMBRYOSCOPY

Embryoscopy is the use of a telescope-like instrument which is passed either into the vagina and through the cervix or through the abdominal wall to provide direct visualization of the fetus. It is used in the first three months of pregnancy and provides spectacular moving pictures of the fetus. It is currently used largely as a research tool in several specialized centres. There have been difficulties in developing good equipment. To view the fetus the outside membrane around it must be ruptured. There is concern that by rupturing the outside sac there may be unacceptable risk to the pregnancy, so it is not yet in widespread use. If the risks can be shown to be low it may well evolve into a useful technique.

INTRAUTERINE TREATMENT

Treatment of abnormalities before birth has aroused the curiosity and excitement of doctors and scientists in this field for many years. The concept of detecting an abnormality and then treating it to allow the delivery of a healthy baby must be the goal of any test in pregnancy. In this short section all that can be done is introduce the concepts of treatment and briefly describe conditions that may be treated. It must be appreciated that very few abnormalities can be treated before birth.

The first and most straightforward method of treatment before birth is to give the pregnant woman a drug which will cross the placenta to the fetus. This method has been used for many years to mature the lungs prior to an anticipated premature birth; if steroids are given to the pregnant woman they cross the placenta and result in the fetus producing a fluid which lines the air cavities of the lungs and stops them collapsing after birth. Drugs may also be given to the pregnant woman if the fetal heartbeat is irregular to help regulate it.

The most successful direct treatment of complications prior to birth is blood transfusion. It is most commonly used where there is incompatibility between the blood of the fetus and the pregnant woman, resulting in the red blood cells of the fetus being destroyed. The fetus can become very anaemic, its tissues become swollen with fluid, and it can ultimately die. Injection of blood into the fetus will prevent this happening and usually allow the delivery of a healthy baby. The blood may be injected into the fetal abdomen and be slowly absorbed into its circulation or it may be injected directly into one of the blood vessels, usually in the umbilical cord. While these procedures may be technically difficult, in expert hands they will result in a high percentage of babies who would have otherwise died being delivered normal and healthy.

Other methods of direct treatment of the fetus have been less successful, but include treatment for hydrocephaly (water on the brain), hydronephrosis (blocked outflow from the kidneys), and fluid in the cavity around the lungs (hydrothorax). These conditions result in a large collection of fluid, which builds up in the affected area. Many such fetuses have been treated by placing a tube, called a shunt, with one end in the fluid collection and the other in the surrounding amniotic cavity. The drainage of such fluid collections may be technically successful, but often there has been such severe damage to the underlying organs that the baby has little or no chance of healthy survival after birth. Disappointing results have caused the virtual abandonment of treatment of hydrocephaly. A small group of those fetuses with hydrothorax or blocked kidneys who are otherwise normal benefit from a drainage procedure.

The final method of treatment we will discuss is a surgical operation on a fetus. This requires making an incision into the abdomen of the pregnant women, opening the uterus and partially removing the fetus. There are several centres in the world where this is being carried out for procedures such as inserting a shunt or repairing a hernia in the diaphragm. There is still a large amount to be learnt both in selecting which fetuses would benefit from such an operation and in minimizing the risks to the pregnant woman, both in this and subsequent pregnancies. It is uncertain whether such operations will ever be in more widespread use.

Which Tests are Right for You?

chapter 12

Selecting the prenatal tests that are right for you need not be confusing. Women under 35 years of age are normally offered an ultrasound examination at 18 to 20 weeks, and maternal serum screening is also available. Those older than 35 commonly elect to exclude chromosome abnormalities by having an amniocentesis or CVS, as well as an 18–20-week ultrasound. Women aged 35 and older who wish to avoid tests with a risk of miscarriage, and opt for non-invasive, but less accurate, tests for chromosomal abnormality, may have the serum screening test and early ultrasound. This chapter provides an easy reference by summarizing the place of each test.

Testing the fetus for abnormalities is an area of medical diagnosis which began as recently as the 1970s, with the introduction of amniocentesis and primitive ultrasound systems into clinical practice. Technology has advanced to produce a confusing array of tests, and deciding which tests are appropriate can be a daunting task even for the most informed couples. Prenatal tests include:
(i)   ultrasound (at various stages of pregnancy);
(ii) maternal serum screening;
(iii) amniocentesis; and
(iv) CVS.

Prenatal testing is based around the detection of three different types of abnormalities:
(i)   Physical or structural abnormalities: ultrasound, commonly in the middle stages of pregnancy, is used to detect physical defects such as spina bifida, missing limbs or fingers, and abnormalites of internal organs such as the heart, kidneys, and brain.
(ii) Chromosome abnormalities (of which Down syndrome is the commonest and most important): chromosomes are usually tested by either amniocentesis or CVS. Other tests, which do not test the chromosomes themselves, but which may indicate

an increased risk of chromosome abnormality, include maternal serum screening, ultrasound at 10 to 13 weeks, and ultrasound at 18 to 20 weeks.

(iii) Rare abnormalities: there are tests available for those few couples who are at increased risk of a particular abnormality, often because they have previously had an affected baby. These include hundreds of inherited conditions, such as fragile X (a form of intellectual impairment), cystic fibrosis, and thalassemia.

PHYSICAL OR STRUCTURAL ABNORMALITIES

Ultrasound at 18 to 20 weeks

An ultrasound examination at this time allows accurate assessment of the age of the pregnancy, identification of the site of the placenta, and diagnosis of multiple pregnancy and of many structural abnormalities. In low-risk women who have had a previously regular menstrual cycle, and who were not on the oral contraceptive pill, the main benefit of an ultrasound examination at this time is to check for fetal abnormalities. It follows that maximum benefit is derived if the scan is carried out at an experienced centre that sees large numbers of pregnant women and is therefore skilled at detecting fetal abnormality. If the scan is carried out at an inexperienced centre that is less likely to detect abnormalities, there is less benefit in having the examination.

Earlier Ultrasound Examination

All of the structures of the fetus that are examined at 18 to 20 weeks can usually be seen at around 13 weeks, given good ultrasound equipment and access to a vaginal ultrasound transducer. It follows that most of the abnormalities that can be detected at 18 to 20 weeks can also be detected at this earlier time. Because the fetus is much smaller, however, the detection is more difficult and, if technical difficulties arise, may be impossible, so a scan at this early time does not replace a scan at 18 to 20 weeks.

If you have a special concern about physical abnormality you may choose to have an ultrasound examination at around 13 weeks, as well as the routine examination offered at 18 to 20 weeks. This allows couples with particular concerns, or who have previously had a baby with a structural abnormality, to be reassured much earlier in the pregnancy. In general, however, unless there was some specific risk, or a high level of anxiety, it would not be considered worth having an additional scan at this early time.

Serum Screening Tests

These blood tests screen for spina bifida as well as for Down syndrome. One of the substances tested for is alpha-fetoprotein (AFP), which occurs in high levels in the pregnant woman's blood in about 90 per cent of anencephalic pregnancies and 85 per cent of spina bifida pregnancies. A raised AFP indicates that there is an increased risk of spina bifida or anencephaly being present, but most women with a positive test result will deliver normal, healthy babies. If the level is raised, the next step is an ultrasound examination to check the dates, because the interpretation of the result depends on the precise number of weeks of pregnancy. Since ultrasound can detect over 95 per cent of fetuses with spina bifida, and all of those with anencephaly, if the ultrasound examination is normal there is a very low chance of either abnormality being present.

Spina bifida can also be diagnosed using amniocentesis, but most couples whose fetus is at increased risk of spina bifida decide not to have an amniocentesis if the spine appears normal on ultrasound examination.

CHROMOSOME ABNORMALITIES

Prenatal tests for Down syndrome (and other chromosome abnormalities) fit into one of two categories: those designed to detect all affected fetuses, and those designed to detect only some. Because Down syndrome is the most common chromosome abnormality, and is also the most common cause of intellectual impairment, it is usually the focus of discussions of chromosome abnormality.

Tests That Detect All Cases of Down Syndrome

The two commonly used tests that will diagnose virtually all cases of chromosome abnormality, including Down syndrome, are amniocentesis, carried out at 15 to 17 weeks, and CVS, carried out any time after 10 weeks. If you wish to have a test for Down syndrome you will need to choose between amniocentesis, which carries a miscarriage rate of about one in 200, or CVS, which is carried out earlier but has a slightly higher miscarriage rate of up to one in 100. These tests are discussed in detail in chapters 6 and 7.

Tests That Detect Some Cases of Down Syndrome

The two tests that allow detection of some fetuses with Down syndrome are ultrasound at 10 to 13 weeks, ultrasound at 18 to 20 weeks, and maternal serum screening.

Ultrasound

Many fetuses with Down syndrome and other chromosome abnormalities have a subtle fluid swelling at the back of the neck at around 10 to 13 weeks, which is known as nuchal oedema. In more than six out of ten fetuses with Down syndrome, this fluid layer is 3 mm or more in thickness at 10 to 13 weeks. Since this fluid tends to absorb, and is therefore no longer detectable at 18 to 20 weeks, an earlier ultrasound examination will detect more cases of Down syndrome. If nuchal oedema is detected, a CVS is offered.

As mentioned above, an ultrasound examination at 18 to 20 weeks is less likely to detect fetuses with Down syndrome. However, even at this stage, some fetuses with Down syndrome will show suspicous signs on careful examination, in which case a sample of amniotic fluid, placenta, or fetal blood can be taken to test the chromosomes. Widely varying claims have been made for the accuracy of ultrasound detection of Down syndrome at 18 to 20 weeks, but most practitioners have been disappointed at the small numbers detected.

Serum Screening Tests

A blood sample is taken from the pregnant woman and three or more substances are measured and analysed in relation to the age of the woman (see chapter 8). If the result shows that the risk of Down syndrome is higher than one in 250, amniocentesis is offered. This blood test detects approximately 60 to 80 per cent of Down syndrome fetuses. Results vary depending on exactly what the laboratory measures and whether the dates are first checked with ultrasound.

The results of maternal serum screening are better when there is a statewide program, so that laboratories are dealing with large numbers of specimens and their level of experience is increased. It is, however, also available through private laboratories.

RARE ABNORMALITIES

Couples with concerns about the risk of particular abnormalities occurring should discuss them with their doctor, who may refer them to a geneticist if the problem is complex.

A SIMPLE GUIDE TO PRENATAL TESTS

When you are considering which tests are appropriate for your pregnancy, it is important to be aware of which risk factors, if any, apply in your situation. The following will help you decide.

Couples at Increased Risk

(i) Age 35+ and wish to undergo testing for chromosome abnormality:

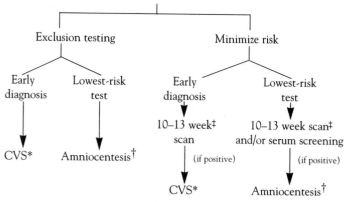

Exclusion testing

Minimize risk

Early diagnosis → CVS*

Lowest-risk test → Amniocentesis†

Early diagnosis → 10–13 week‡ scan → (if positive) → CVS*

Lowest-risk test → 10–13 week scan‡ and/or serum screening → (if positive) → Amniocentesis†

18–20-week scan — as for couples at low risk (see p. 178)

* Termination of pregnancy performed by simple curette.
† Termination of pregnancy mostly performed by induced labour.
‡ Detection rate depends on experience of operator.

(ii) Previous abnormality: Couples who have previously had a baby with an abnormality will be anxious about a recurrence. If the abnormality was structural, an ultrasound examination at around 13 weeks allows early diagnosis, but remember this does not replace an ultrasound scan at 18 to 20 weeks.

(iii) Other specific abnormalities: *These require individual consideration.*

Couples at Low Risk

(i)   Under 35 with no other risk factors:

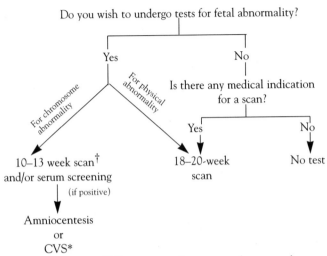

Do you wish to undergo tests for fetal abnormality?

Yes — No

For chromosome abnormality / For physical abnormality

Is there any medical indication for a scan?

Yes — No

10–13 week scan† and/or serum screening

18–20-week scan

No test

(if positive)

Amniocentesis or CVS*

* Amniocentesis or CVS are options for women of any age who are particularly concerned, but few under 35 request these tests without a positive ultrasound or serum screening test.

† Detection rate depends on experience of operator.

THE FUTURE OF PRENATAL DIAGNOSIS

As screening programs become available using ultrasound at 10 to 13 weeks, and serum screening in the third month, fewer women are likely to have CVS or amniocentesis because of their age alone. Since measurement techniques vary, well-organized, centralized programs will be required if results are to be relied upon. The risk of Down syndrome could be calculated by combining the pregnant woman's age, ultrasound at 10 to 13 weeks, and an early serum screening test. This would allow couples to make an informed decision on testing by 10 weeks of pregnancy.

Although most detectable physical abnormalities can be seen on ultrasound at 13 weeks, a scan will continue to be offered to all pregnant women at 18 to 20 weeks because at this stage of pregnancy it is easier to see and record all the fetal structures.

A. Clegg, A. Woolett, *Twins: From Conception to Five Years*, First Ballantine Books, New York 1988.

M. A. England, *A Colour Atlas of Life Before Birth: Normal Fetal Development*, Wolfe Medical Publications, London, 1983.

J. Fletcher, D. Wertz, Ethical aspects of prenatal diagnosis: Views of U.S. medical geneticists, *Clinics in Perinatology*, 1987 14, 293–312.

R. J. M. Gardner and G. R. Sutherland, *Chromosome Abnormalities and Genetic Counselling*, 2nd edn, Oxford University Press, Oxford, 1996.

H. Kuhse and P. Singer, *Should the Baby Live?*, Oxford University Press, Oxford, 1985.

J. H. Lord, *No Time for Goodbyes: Coping with Sorrow, Anger and Injustice after a Tragic Death*, Pathfinder, Ventura, CA, 1987.

L. McCullough and F. Chervenate, *Ethics in Obstetrics and Gynecology*, Oxford University Press, New York, 1994.

R. Romero, G. Pilu, P. Jeanty, A. Ghidini, J. Hobbins, *Prenatal Diagnosis of Congenital Abnormalities*, Appleton & Lange, Connecticut 1988.

B. K. Rothman, *The Tentative Pregnancy: Prenatal Diagnosis and the Future of Motherhood*, Viking, New York, 1986.

M. J. Schleifer and S. D. Klein, *The Disabled Child and the Family: An Exceptional Parent Reader*, Exceptional Parent Press, Boston, 1985.

Simons, R. *After the Tears: Parents Talk About Raising a Child with a Disability*, Harcourt Brace Jovanovich, San Diego, 1987.

P. Singer, *Rethinking Life and Death*, Text Publishing Co., Melbourne, 1994.

Introduction
L. de Crespigny, 'Standards of mid-trimester ultrasound in Australia',
 MJA 1995, 163, 31–2.

Chapter 1
R. E. Scammon, and L. A. Calkins, *The Development and Growth of
 the External Dimensions of the Human Body in the Fetal Period*,
 University of Minnesota Press, Minneapolis, 1929.

B. K. Rothman, *The Tentative Pregnancy: Prenatal Diagnosis and the
 Future of Motherhood*, Viking, New York, 1986.

Chapter 2
D. Cox, B. Wittmann, M. Hess et al., 'The psychological impact of
 diagnostic ultrasound', *Obstet Gynecol* 1987, 70, 673–6.

G. R. de Vore, 'The routine antenatal diagnostic imaging with ultrasound study: Another perspective', *Obstet Gynecol* 1994, 84,
 622–6.

B. G. Ewigman, J. P. Crane, F. D. Frigoletto et al., 'Effect of prenatal
 ultrasound screening on perinatal outcome', *N Engl J Med* 1993,
 329, 821–7.

A. Saari-Kemppainen, O. Karjalainen, P. Ylostalo, O. Heinonen,
 'Ultrasound screening and perinatal mortality: Controlled trial of
 systematic one-stage screening in pregnancy', *Lancet* 1990, 386,
 387–91.

S. B. Thacker, 'Quality of controlled clinical trials. The case of imaging ultrasound in obstetrics; a review', *Br J Obstet Gynaecol* 1985,
 92, 437–44

Chapter 3
M. B. Braken, 'Ultrasonography in antenatal management: Should it
 be a routine procedure?', *Fetal Ther* 1987, 20, 2–6.

D. Liebeskind, R. Bases, F. Mendez et al., 'Sister chromatid exchanges
 in human lymphocytes after exposure to diagnostic ultrasound',
 Science 1979, 205, 1273–5.

W. McDonald, J. Newnham, L. Gurrin et al. 'Effect of frequent pre-natal ultrasound on birth weight: Follow-up at 1 year of age', *Lancet* 1996, 348, 482.

C. R. Stark, M. Orleans, A. D. Haverkamp, and J. Murphy, 'Short- and long-term risks after exposure to diagnostic ultrasound in utero', *Obstet Gynecol* 1984, 63, 194–200.

L. Warsof and S. K. Sayegh, 'Ultrasound diagnosis of intrauterine growth retardation', *Fetal Ther* 1987, 2, 31–6

Chapter 4

E. Dreazen, F. Tessler, D. Sarti, B. F. Crandall, 'Spontaneous resolution of fetal hydrocephalus', *J Ultrasound Med* 1989, 8, 155–7.

R. Romero, G. Pilu, P. Jeanty, A. Ghidini and J. Hobbins, *Prenatal Diagnosis of Congenital Anomalies*, Appleton & Lange, 1988.

H. Rosendahl, S. Kivinen, 'Antenatal detection of congenital malformations by routine ultrasonography', *Obstet Gynecol* 1989, 73, 947–51.

Chapter 5

M. A. Ferguson-Smith and J. R. W. Yates, 'Maternal age-specific rates for chromosome aberrations and factors influencing them: A report of a collaborative European study on 56,965 amniocenteses', *Prenat Diagn* 1984, 4, 5–44.

T. Fryers *The Epidemiology of Severe Intellectual Impairment*, Academic Press, London, 1984.

R. J. M. Gardner and G. R. Sutherland, *Chromosome Abnormalities and Genetic Counselling*, 2nd edn, Oxford University Press, Oxford, 1996.

J. L. Halliday, L. F. Watson, J. Lumley, et al., 'New estimates of Down syndrome risks at chorionic villus sampling, amniocentesis, and livebirth in women of advanced maternal age from a uniquely defined population', *Prenat Diagn* 1995, 15, 455–65.

B. E. Hashimoti, B. S. Mahony, R. A. Filly, et al., 'Sonography: A complementary examination to alpha-fetoprotein testing for fetal neural tube defects', *J Ultrasound Med*, 1985, 4; 307–10.

E. B. Hook and P. K. Cross, 'Interpretation of recent data pertinent to genetic counselling for Down syndrome: Maternal-age specific rates, temporal trends, adjustments for paternal age, recurrence risks, risks after other cytogenetic abnormalities, recurrence risk after remarriage', in A. M. Willey, T. P. Carter,

S. Kelly and I. H. Porter (eds), *Clinical Genetics: Problems in Diagnosis and Counseling*, Academic Press, New York, 1982, pp. 119–39.

E. B. Hook, P. K. Cross, L. Jackson, E. Pergament and B. Brambati, 'Maternal age-specific rates of 47, +21 and other cytogenetic abnormalities diagnosed in the first trimester of pregnancy in chorionic villus biopsy specimens: Comparison with rates expected from observations at amniocentesis', *Am J Hum Genet* 1988, 42, 797–807.

S. G. Ratcliffe and N. Paul, *Prospective Studies on Children with Sex Chromosome Aneuploidy*, Liss, New York 1986

Chapter 6

B. F. Crandall, J. Howard, T. B. Lebherz et al., 'Follow-up of 2000 second-trimester amniocenteses', *Obstet Gynecol* 1980, 56, 625–8.

L. Ch. de Crespigny and H. P. Robinson, 'Amniocentesis: A comparison of 'monitored' versus 'blind' needle insertion technique', *Aust NZ J Obstet Gynaecol* 1986, 26, 124–8.

B. Elejalde, M. de Elejalde, J. M. Acunda et al., 'Prospective study of amniocentesis performed between weeks 9 and 16 of gestation', *Am J Med Genet* 1990, 35, 188–96.

K. P. Katayama and M. R. Roesler, 'Five hundred cases of amniocentesis without bloody tap', *Obstet Gynecol* 1986, 68, 70–3.

W. F. O'Brien, 'Midtrimester genetic amniocentesis. A review of fetal risks', *J Reprod Med* 1984, 29, 59–63.

L. Pijpers, M. G. Jahoda, R. P. Vosters et al., 'Genetic amniocentesis in twin pregnancies', *Br J Obstet Gynaecol* 1988, 95, 323–326.

A. Tabor, J. Philip, M. Madsen et al., 'Randomised controlled trial of genetic amniocentesis in 4606 low-risk women', *Lancet* 1986, 1, 1287–93.

M. Verjaal and N. J. Leschot, 'Risk of amniocentesis and laboratory findings in a series of 1500 prenatal diagnoses', *Prenat Diagn* 1981, 1, 173–81.

R. A. Williamson, M. W. Varner, S. S. Grant, 'Reduction in amniocentesis risks using a real-time needle guide procedure', *Obstet Gynecol* 1985, 65, 751–5.

Chapter 7

A. Boogert, A. Mantingh and G. Visser, 'The immediate effects of chorionic villus sampling on fetal movements', *Am J Obstet Gynecol*, 1987, 157, 137–9.

B. Brambati, A. Lanzani and L. Tului, 'Transabdominal and transcervical chorionic villus sampling: Efficiency and risk evaluation of 2411 cases', *Am J Med Genet* 1990, 35, 160–4.

B. Brambati, L. Tului, G. Simoni and M. Travi, 'Prenatal diagnosis at six weeks', *Lancet* 1988, 2, 397.

Canadian Collaborative CVS-Amniocentesis Clinical Trial Group, 'Multicentre randomised clinical trial of chorion villus sampling and amniocentesis', *Lancet* 1989, 1, 1–6.

L. de Crespigny, H. Robinson and A. Ngu, 'Pain with amniocenfitesis and transabdominal CVS', *Aust NZ J Obstet Gynaecol* 1990, 30, 308–9.

A. G. Hunter, H. Muggah, B. Ivey, D. M. Cox, 'Assessment of the early risks of chorionic villus sampling', *Can Med Assoc J* 1986, 134, 753–6.

L. Jackson, 'CVS latest news', Division of Medical Genetics, Jefferson Medical College, Philadelphia, May 1990, No. 28.

A. Kuliev, B. Modell, L. Jackson, 'Risk evaluation of CVS', *Prenat Diagn* 1993, 13, 197–209.

G. Monni, G. Olla and A. Cao, 'Patients' choice between transcervical and transabdominal chorionic villus sampling', *Lancet* 1988, 1, 1057.

G. C. Rhoads, L. G. Jackson, S. E. Schlesselman et al., 'The safety and efficacy of chorionic villus sampling for early prenatal diagfinosis of cytogenetic abnormalities', *N Engl J Med* 1989, 320, 609–17.

G. Robinson, D. Garner, M. Olmsted et al., 'Anxiety reduction after chorionic villus sampling and genetic amniocentesis', *AMJ Obstet Gynecol* 1988, 159, 953–6.

H. P. Robinson, L. de Crespigny, A. Ngu et al., 'Transabdominal chorionic villus sampling: A safe and reliable procedure'. In press.

J. Spencer and D. Cox, 'A comparison of chorionic villi sampling and amniocentesis: Acceptability of procedure and maternal attachment to pregnancy', *Obstet Gynecol* 1988, 72 714–17.

Chapter 8

T. M. Marleav et al., 'The psychological effects of false-positive results in prenatal testing for fetal abnormality: A prospective study', *Prenat Diagn* 1992, 12, 205–14.

R. J. M. Snij   ders, S. Johnson, N. J. Sebire et al., 'First trimester ultrasound screening for chromosomal defects', *Ultrasound in Obstet Gynecol* 1996, 7,

216–26.

N. Wald, H. Cuckle, J. Densem et al., 'Maternal serum screening for Down's syndrome in early pregnancy', *Br Med J* 1988, 297, 883–7.

S. C. Yeoh, I. L. Sargent, C. W. G. Redman and S. L. Thein, 'Detecting fetal cells in maternal circulation', *Lancet* 1989, 2, 869–70.

Chapter 9

P. Singer, *Rethinking Life and Death*, Text Publishing Co., Melbourne, 1994.

L. Skene, 'Prentatal diagnosis and late termination', *Aust NZ J Obstet Gynaecol* 1995, 35, 3–6.

D. Wertz and J. Fletcher, 'Ethical problems in prenatal diagnosis: A cross-cultural survey of medical geneticists in 18 nations', *Prenat Diagn* 1989, 9, 145–57.

Chapter 10

Keeley & Bean (eds), *Australian Attitudes*, Allen & Unwin, Sydney, 1988.

Tabor et al., ibid.

Spencer and Cox, ibid.

Robinson et al., ibid.

S. L. Clark and G. R. DeVore, 'Prenatal diagnosis for couples who would not consider abortion', *Obstet Gynecol* 1989, 73, 1035–7.

Chapter 11

ACOG Committee Opinion, 'Guidelines for diagnostic imaging during pregnancy', *Int J Obstet Gynecol* 1995, 51, 288–91.

P. Boulot, F. Deschamps, G. Lefort et al., 'Pure fetal blood samples obtained by cordocentesis: Technical aspects of 322 cases', *Prenat Diagn* 1990, 10, 93–100.

F. Daffos, M. Capella-Pavlowsky, F. Forestier, 'Fetal blood sampling during pregnancy with use of a needle guided by ultrasound, a study of 606 consecutive cases', *Am J Obstet Gynecol* 1985, 153, 655–60.

M. J. Whittle, 'Cordocentesis', *Br J Obstet Gynaecol* 1989, 96, 262–4.